Real Answers

Prostate Cancer

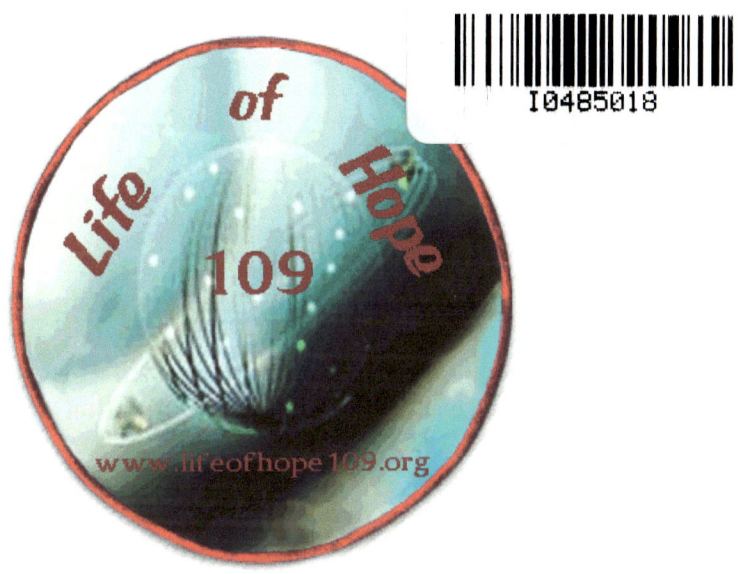

The Real Questions Men Don't Like To Talk About

Proceeds and Donations go to help men who can't
afford treatments or other help with Prostate Cancer.

DEDICATION

Dr. Paul D. Silverman and Dr. Marc A Beaghler

Adult & Pediatric Urology's.

All Prostate Cancer Patience's and Survivors of Prostate Cancer and all my friends and family for their prayers and Support.

Awareness

Increase by 2010 awareness of prostate cancer risk factors as well as the benefits and risks of prostate cancer screening among primary care physicians, high-risk men, and the general public.

Objectives

• [4]By 2010, there will be a 30% increase in knowledge of the 2006 Michigan Cancer Consortium prostate cancer early detection recommendations among primary care physicians (Baseline 1995 KAP surveys), the public, and high-risk populations (Baseline 1995 KAP surveys; SCBRFSS 2001-02).
• By 2010, increase from 70% to 80% the awareness of prostate cancer risk factors among African American men.
• By 2010, there will be a 30% increase in adherence to the 2005 Michigan Cancer Consortium Prostate Cancer Early Detection Recommendations* among primary care physicians, with particular emphasis on populations of higher than average prostate cancer risk.

All References, Graphics use by Permission.
Co Authors: Paul D. Silverman, M.D., Duke K. Bahn, M.D.

The mission of Life of Hope 109 Support Groups for Men and Women is to provide a safe and emotionally supportive network for all; regardless of race, religion or creed.

Publish by: Life of Hope 109 = http://www.lifeofhope109.org

Information or Questions: EMail Jerry at: hope@lifeofhope109.org

Content: Page:

Real Answers

The Real Questions Men Don't Like To Talk About

1. Sex Life

2. Saving the Nerves

3. Pads for men

4. The Catheter

5. Recovery Time = Depends on the procedural you decide on

6. Be Cheerful, Have Hope, Prayer and Faith

7. Talk to Family and Friends

8. ED = Erection

9. Join A Support Group

10. The Biopsy

11. PSA Test

12. Your Treatment

According to the American Cancer Society, prostate cancer is the most commonly occurring cancer in males today and is number two cause in cancer-related death in men, ahead of colon cancer and second only to lung cancer.

Prostate Cancer will affect one out of every five men during their lifetime—it is the second most common cancer in men. The American Cancer Society estimates that 189,000 new cases will be detected in the United States each year. It is more common in men after the age of 50 and among men who are African American or have a father or brother who have the disease.

Risk Factors

Men with a family history of prostate cancer are considered to be at high risk. Research suggests that high dietary fat is also a prominent risk factor. There may be a hereditary factor, but no gene has been identified.

Other possible risk factors include the following:

- Age (96 percent of cases occur in men over 55)
- Exposure to heavy metals (e.g., cadmium)
- Infectious agents
- Low exposure to ultraviolet light
- Race (African American men have the highest rate)
- Smoking
- Farmers (probably due to pesticide use)
- Airline pilots
- Vietnam veteran

Screening Prostate Cancer

Prostate cancer screening is an attempt to identify individuals with prostate cancer in a broad segment of the population—those for whom there is no reason to suspect prostate cancer. There are currently two methods used: One is the digital rectal examination (DRE), in which the examiner inserts a gloved, lubricated finger into the rectum to examine the adjoining prostate. The other is the prostate-specific antigen (PSA) blood test, which measures the concentration of this molecule in the blood.

A major question for any screening protocol is how many men will have needless treatment for each man whose life would be saved.

Staging Prostate Cancer

Staging is the assessment of the size and location of prostate cancer (that is, how far the cancer has already spread). Staging is necessary for you and your physician to decide what type of treatment is most appropriate.

Currently, two different systems are used to stage prostate cancer. The traditional method classifies the disease into 4 clinical categories rated A through D. The second system is called TNM, which stands for tumor-nodes-metastases.

Although TNM is the more accepted staging system, the A-D system is stilled used. (see figure 1-L and figures A-D Staging below)

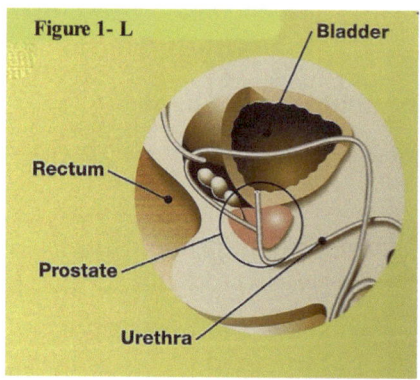

Figure 1- L

Bladder

Rectum

Prostate

Urethra

A–D Staging

Stage A ● is early cancer. The tumor is located within the prostate gland and cannot be detected by a DRE.[9]

In **Stage B,** ● the tumor is considered to be within the prostate but is large enough to be felt during a DRE.[9]

In **Stage C,** ● prostate cancer is more advanced. Stage C indicates that the tumor has spread outside the prostate to some surrounding areas, but has not spread to other organs. This stage of prostate cancer can usually be detected by a DRE.[9]

In **Stage D,** ● the cancer has spread to the nearby organs and usually to distant sites, such as the bones or lymph nodes.[9]

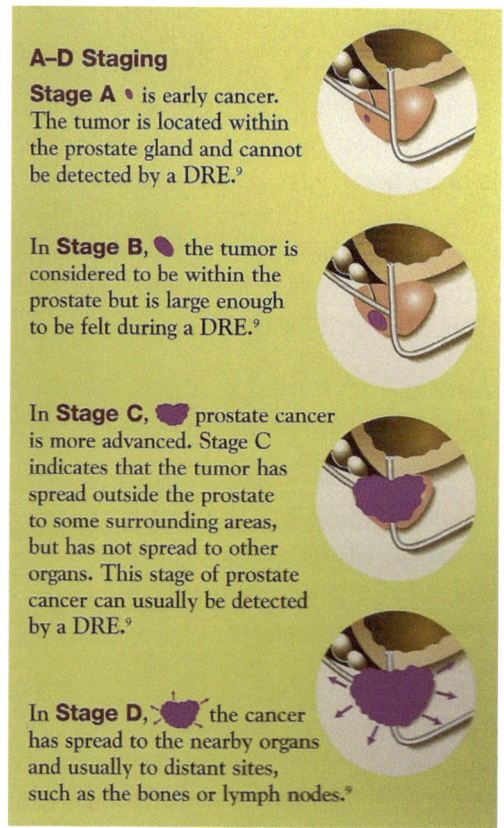

What Men Don't Like To Talk About

A. Most men are embarrass to speak the truth about their sex life.

B. Men over the age of 40 mostly keep their sex life to themselves.

C. While the younger men will only boost to a friend or other men chatting about sex.

Why saying "NO" to sex the night before your PSA test might just save your life... and other things you probably don't know about your prostate health, but should!

No matter what your prostate problem may be...

No matter if you've been diagnosed with prostate cancer...

Even if you think your prostate's just fine for now...

Here's vital information you simply can't afford to ignore.

Did you know...

Having sex within 72 hours of your PSA test can produce a false reading?

Erectile dysfunction can be a symptom of prostate cancer?

About 50% of men over 50 suffer from the life-changing symptoms of an enlarged prostate (BPH), increasing to almost 90% among men over age 80?

About Prostate Cancer

"...prostate cancer accounts for 36% of all male cancers in the United States and 13% of all cancer related deaths in men..."

Adenocarcinoma of the prostate is the clinical term for cancer that begins in the glandular structure of the prostate. If identified while it is confined within the prostate, the cancer can be treated successfully.

The longer prostate cancer is ignored, the greater the chance that it will metastasize (spread), first locally to tissues around the prostate, or seminal vesicles (saclike structures attached to the prostate), then to other parts of the body, such as lymph nodes, bones, liver and lungs.

Prostate cancer is becoming an increasingly important public health concern. The second leading cause of cancer death in men in the United States, its impact is roughly equivalent to the affects of breast cancer on women. Cancer of the prostate is the most common form of malignancy in men—approximately one in nine will develop the disease. In spite of this alarming fact, many men are unaware of the dangers, and the lack of immediate symptoms creates a false sense of security.

Early detection and intervention of progressive prostate cancer may help decrease the 40,000 prostate cancer-related deaths each year. Treated in its early stages, prostate cancer is highly survivable.

Exercise helps, especially in older men. Learn how men 65 and older were able to reduce their risk of advanced prostate cancer by nearly 70%. (see page 78)

Foods that may reduce your risk of prostate cancer.

How your weight can increase your risk of prostate cancer.

D. If you have Prostate Cancer beware, most RN's and LVN's at your Urologist appointment: (Most nurses or assistants will be Women....

Also at your hospital stay the chances of having a male RN is a little on the rare side, but more men are being seen.)

E. Remember they are pros and have seen a man's private parts many, many times.

So just go with the flow.

F. If you are married have your wife with you for support, the only time she will not be allowed is during the rectal exam (most doctors don't allow your support person when you have your biopsy, surgery and removal of the catheter - removal of the stables or stitching of the surgical incisions).

G. Talk to your Urologist about saving the nerves. (for erection) This does depend on what stage you are at, age and other health issues.

H. Ask Questions on issues of pads for men, 5mg of Cialis Viagra, Pumps, Injections, and so on.... Know your Gleason score, PSA level, and tell your doctor to speak up and tell you all your options.

I. Talk to your wife or support person on all issues. Be HONEST on how you feel about any procedurals.

J. After, if you chose to have your prostate removed I do recommend to eat Pitted Prunes, (8-10) every morning, this helps you to have a regular BM until you are fully recovered.

K. As males (Especially T-type Alpha males!) we all tend to be over protective to our sexual packaging--but when the choice comes down to; "quality of life", death or good sex--one has to make that decision themselves as to what is more important.

If you were given advise for treatment by a Urologist, I would advise that you seek out a Prostate Oncologist for a second opinion. This is a unique specialty and worth the effort.

My comment that you need to do your homework, and don't get pushed into any treatment just because of what one doctor says - the old "doctor's agenda" can really put you into a position that you may regret. PLEASE - get on the internet and contact the American Cancer Society. Yes, it's a lot of work, and you might feel that you are becoming more confused by the day from all the information, but it will pay big dividends in the long run.

Very few people are really in the position that the treatment is one of two choices and that's all. Find a urologist in the largest hospital close by and let them review your case.

We are all uniquely different to some degree and in so many ways; our blood type; genetic make up; physical and mental tolerance; our metabolism, and so on. So it becomes difficult to say what is actually best for one as there are no "one-fit-all' solutions.

Every diagnosis and doctor is different, 2nd and 3rd opinions are critical as is your knowledge.

Very few people are really in the position that the treatment is one of two choices and that's all.

Find a urologist in the largest hospital close by and let them review your case. At a Gleason of 6 or 7 appears that time might be on your side as far as getting a second opinion - but don't put off treatment!! (see page 64)

Do a good search for information, ask some good questions of the urologists, and don't let them tell you that there is only one (or two) choices (or make them tell you why - they are working for YOU and they should be willing to answer all your questions.)

Its Okay if you are scared!
After all it is Cancer!

Do you trust your Urologist? You defiantly need to!

You may want to get a second opinion about the best treatment option for your situation, especially if there are several choices available to you.

Tell your doctor you would like to speak to a Cancer Specialist.

How to get your answer from a specialist

Remember they can't tell you what to do!

Be sure to give the Dr. all the procedures you are thinking about.

Don't ask him for his opinion, instead ask him:

(If your were in my position what procedure would you take)

When I went to see my Urologist after my biopsy for my report, my wife and I was waiting in the little room they put you in until the doctor comes in, when he came in he said (Lets go to my office) I knew right then the news was not going to be good.

NOTE: Ask your urologist for copies of your report, its your right to see and have a copy of your actual results.

My wife took it a lot harder than me! We didn't talk very much on the way home about the situation.

When we got home we talked about my situation, I went on the internet and started reading every thing I could fine on Prostate Cancer, I join a online support group and received lots of feedback and help.

See: http://www.lifeofhope109.org and join in.

I have done a very intensive research on Prostate Cancer and talked to many, many doctors, cancer specialist and they all said (if I was in your place I would go with the da Vinci Robotic surgery) My opinion this is the way to go, If you have that option.

This is base on your age and your overall health. It's a long procedure about 4 1/2 to 5 1/2 hours.

If I had to do it all over again, I would not think twice about having the da Vince Robotic Surgery again.

Keep a positive attitude, Have Faith, Hope and Prayer

I only had one moment on Wednesday night a week before my surgery I got scared, and I talked to my wife about the problem and she was a big help, Please don't be afraid to speak about having Prostate Cancer.

From that moment on I never had a negative thought.

The day of my surgery I was happy and cheerful and didn't think twice about what was going to take place. I had Faith in God and my doctors and I knew everything was going to be fine.

A quote from my support page: Jerry L. Mayers

I have had my da Vince robotic surgery and I'm doing Great! I never had to take any Pain meds when I was in the hospital, I went home that Friday morning, The only thing I took was a prescription Tylenol for a little pain.

I had NO TROUBLE.

I had a fast recovery and The surgeon was able to save my nerves. It took less than 4 weeks to fully recover and I'm doing great! I have full control over my urination.

All I can say is in my suggestion that the da Vince Robotic is the Best way to go. My report is now I'm CANCER FREE.

THANKS to my Support Group, Friends, my Doctors, my Wife and Family for the Support and Prayers.

Jerry L Mayers

My Surgery Videos:

Websites: Copy and paste into your browser.

http://www.youtube.com/jlmayers46 Main Site two parts.

There are many treatment options for prostate cancer, and new treatment options are here NOW.

Get to know your prognosis and understand your treatment options before choosing a course of action.

A Battle Between the Immune System and Cancer

As most of us know, the immune system plays a critical role in controlling and eliminating infectious organisms, including many bacteria and viruses. More controversial has been the question of whether the immune system can effectively control cancer growth and metastases. The last several years have provided new insights into how the immune system works, along with possible means to activate the system so that immune cells will recognize markers on cancer cells and destroy these cells. These advances have led to the emergence of a new and promising therapeutic strategy in cancer treatment, referred to as tumor immunotherapy, which can successfully treat and possibly cure selected patients.[1,2]

A potentially key weapon is the dendritic cell (DC), a scarce white blood cell that can now be generated by the millions in the laboratory, where they are cultured from precursor cells that circulate in the blood. Dendritic cells are the body's scavengers, constantly prowling our bodies in an effort to communicate to the immune system the various biological goings-on in the cells throughout the body. In the case of disease states involving bacteria, virally infected cells, and cancer cells, distinct molecular markers, called antigens, reveal the problematic nature of these cells.

Dendritic cells gobble up these cells and break them down into smaller protein fragments which they prominently display on their cell surfaces (Figure 1). The dendritic cells then migrate to the nearest lymph node, rather like detectives returning with evidence to the forensic lab at the local precinct station, in this case bringing biochemical evidence of disease with them.

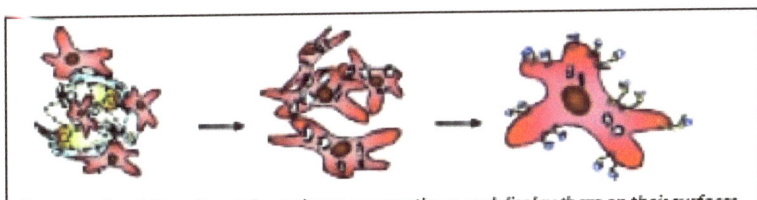
Figure 1. Dendritic cells uptake antigens, process them, and display them on their surfaces.

In the lymph node, the dendritic cells present the biochemical evidence to lymphocytes known as "naïve T cells" (Figure 2).

If the presented antigen is identified as "problematic" – i.e. related to infection or cancer – certain naïve T cells are capable of undergoing activation, wherein their numbers increase greatly. These activated T cells migrate out of the lymph node and search the body for cells bearing the same antigens and kill them (Figure 2). Among these T cells are the same type of killer T cells that will attack and unleash torrents of strikingly powerful substances in an attack that can completely destroy organs weighing several pounds (such as the kidney, liver, or heart) in mismatched human transplants.

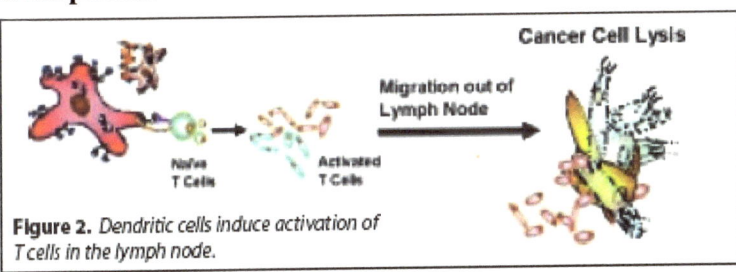
Figure 2. Dendritic cells induce activation of T cells in the lymph node.

Strategies using dendritic cells to fight cancer (dendritic cell vaccination) have entered clinical testing in the past decade.[3] Most of these methods administer patients' own dendritic cells after first "arming" them with a synthetic cancer antigen in the laboratory. Patients' T cells specific for the chosen cancer antigen are activated and can in theory kill cancer cells bearing the antigen (Figure 3).

These studies have shown that dendritic cell injections were well tolerated with minimal side effects. Clinical responses were observed in approximately half of the trials.[4]

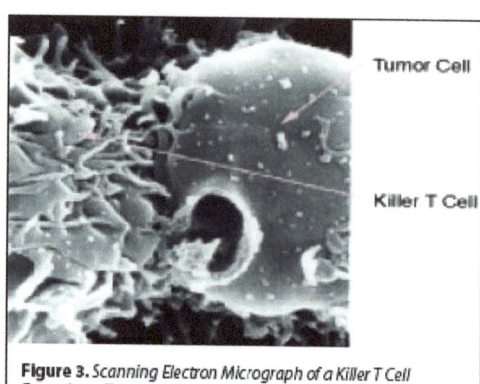

Figure 3. *Scanning Electron Micrograph of a Killer T Cell Engaging a Tumor Cell.*

An alternative strategy for dendritic cell vaccination is to introduce a patient's dendritic cells into the cancerous tissue5, thus allowing these dendritic cells to acquire antigens directly from that patient's own cancer cells ("intra-tumoral dendritic cell injection"). Since cancer is generally composed of a heterogeneous (highly variable) population of cancerous cells expressing numerous antigens, multiple cancer antigens can, in theory, be acquired by dendritic cells using this strategy. Vaccines that target multiple antigens may be a superior choice for eliciting a more complete immune response against cancer than those that target only one antigen.

Releasing Antigens from a Tumor

It has been speculated that an even more efficient means of obtaining the antigenic components of a cancerous mass in the body might involve first damaging the tumor - thereby causing it to release some or all of its antigens - and then introducing the dendritic cells into the damaged tumor environment. These dendritic cells may then be able to better acquire the tumor antigens (as in Figure 1) than if the tumor cells had not been damaged before the injection of the dendritic cells into the tumor mass.

This speculation has found support in several recently reported studies. For instance, when mice with implanted experimental tumors were treated with chemotherapy followed by injection of dendritic cells into the growing tumor, complete regression of these tumors was observed.6,7

No such regression was noted when the mice were treated with chemotherapy alone or dendritic cell injection alone. In these cases, chemotherapy hypothetically resulted in cellular death of part of the rapidly growing tumors.

Similar observations have been noted when the "damaging" treatment was hyperthermia (heat)[8], radiation[9], or cryotherapy [10, 11] of the tumor. In these cases, the mice that received the combination of the damaging therapy and the injection of dendritic cells into the damaged tumor fared significantly better – as measured by either the growth of the tumors, the number of new tumors, or the survival of the mice – than the mice that received the damaging treatment or dendritic cell injection alone.

Taken together, these observations suggest that there may be a therapeutic approach to human cancers that combines a tumor damaging strategy followed by the injection of autologous, or self-derived, dendritic cells into the treated tumor. An example of such an approach is a Stanford University clinical trial that damages liver tumors with thermotherapy (heat), followed by dendritic cell injection. [5]

Dendritic Cell-Based Cryo-Immunotherapy

In the spring of 2004, the Seattle-based Haakon Ragde Foundation partnered with Sangretech Biomedical, a Seattle biotech company, and the Prostate Institute of America in Ventura, California, to study a similar immunotherapeutic modality.[12] This therapeutic approach entails the use of cryotherapy (freezing) of prostate tumors followed by intra-tumoral dendritic cell injection. This combination is known as "dendritic cell based cryo-immunotherapy." In this case, tumor damage and antigen liberation is achieved via cryotreatment of the prostate and/or metastases. (See Figure 4.) An investigation of this combination in PC patients is currently underway at the Asian Hospital and Medical Center in Manila, the Philippines.

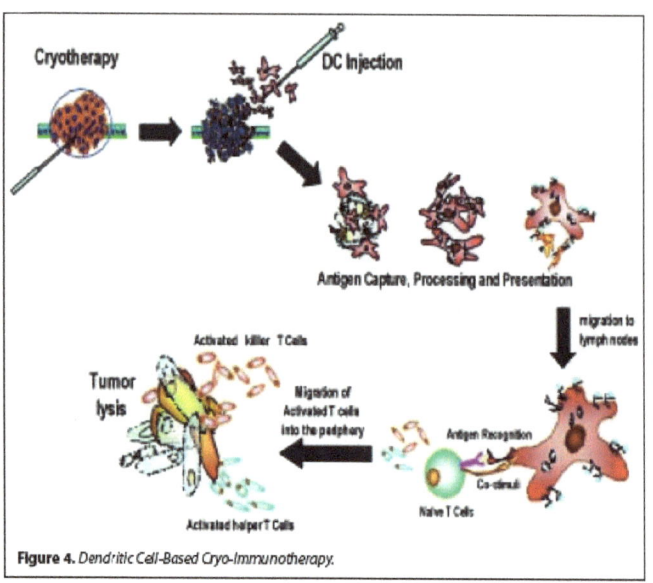

Figure 4. *Dendritic Cell-Based Cryo-Immunotherapy.*

The primary objective of this study is to explore the safety of a potential cancer treatment that first freezes the prostate, and follows with an injection of millions of the patient's own dendritic cells into the gland. As stated above, this process may allow dendritic cells to capture tumor antigens released by the dying PC cells in response to the cryotherapy. As illustrated schematically in Figures 1 and 2, the process is designed to result in a system-wide immune assault upon remaining tumor cells that have spread - or may have spread - from the original, primary PC.

In contrast to other tumor-damaging approaches such as chemotherapy and radiation, cryotherapy may be a superior means of damaging the tumor and releasing tumor antigen. There is strong biological evidence to support this hypothesis: first, cryotherapy will not damage the immune system as chemotherapy and radiation do. Second, it is well established that immunotherapy works best with smaller tumor volumes, and cryo-destruction results in a swift reduction of most of the cancerous mass (along with a predictable release of antigen).

Seven PC patients have traveled to the Philippines to take part in this trial in 2005.

Although additional clinical evidence will be necessary before any conclusions regarding Cryo-Immunotherapy's safety and effectiveness may be reliably ascertained, early labs results (including PSA) in these seven patients are encouraging. Additional labs tests, imaging studies, and physical evaluations in the seven patients treated thus far are ongoing. Based on these early results, a U.S. trial, to take place at the Prostate Institute of America in Ventura, California, is in the planning stages. Studies are also being contemplated in other cancer types, as the technique is applicable in theory to most solid tumor cancer.

No significant toxicity issues related to dendritic cell administration have been encountered to date. Cryoablation of the prostate has led to some common and expected side effects, specifically some fatigue and some non-febrile sweating during the first 24-48 hours after treatment, though these were temporary. Overall, dendritic cell-based cryo-immunotherapy has been well tolerated by the first seven patients.

Therapeutic cancer vaccines are attractive because of their negligible side effects that allow patients to maintain their quality of life – a privilege rarely possible with conventional cancer treatments.

As clinical responses to vaccine therapy continue to advance as a result of new knowledge and improved techniques, there will be an increasing use of this modality in the management of all solid cancers, both for clinically localized cancers and for cancers that have spread.

Early Detection

After more than 30 years of studies and trials and hundreds of millions of dollars, it has been proven that early detection is the only contributing factor for better cancer control and improved survival. Early detection and early intervention of progressive prostate cancer may help to decrease the 40,000 plus prostate cancer-related deaths each year.

All men 45 years or older should have a PSA test (blood test), an annual rectal exam and, if necessary, a transrectal ultrasound (TRUS). Men between the ages of 40 and 49 should have a PSA screening if an immediate family member has prostate cancer or if they are African American.

Early detection and early intervention of progressive prostate cancer may help to decrease the 40,000 plus prostate cancer-related deaths each year. The updated American Cancer Society's recommendations for prostate cancer detection in asymptomatic men are that annual PSA and DRE (digital rectal examination) should be offered to men aged 50 or older who have at least a 10-year life expectancy, and to younger men at higher risk, such as African-American men or men with a strong familiar predisposition to prostate cancer (two or more affected first-degree relatives, e.g., father, brother).

Patients should be given information regarding the potential risks and benefits of intervention.

It is our recommendation that a patient should proceed to a transrectal ultrasound if the PSA level is more than 2.5 ng/ml or the digital rectal examination is abnormal, regardless of the PSA level. For high risk men, an ultrasound examination is recommended if their PSA level is over 2.0 mg/ml.

The Importance of Accurate Diagnosis

Over the past several years, increases in the reported incidence of prostate cancer have been disproportionate to the changes in the population demographics. The main reason for this rapid rise may be the easy access to PSA (blood test)and subsequent ultrasound guided biopsies (random biopsy).

Mass screening efforts present a dilemma for the patients and the clinicians. Although saving many lives, screenings also pick up so called "latent" or "insignificant" tumors that may not need any treatment.

It is reported that 15 to 20 percent of patients who have a radical prostatectomy may have been exposed to unnecessary surgery and related post-surgical complications. Screenings are justifiable and treatments are usually effective when either slow-growing progressive cancers (which will become symptomatic and can kill) or rapidly progressing (very malignant cancers that are likely to kill) are detected. Unfortunately, it is difficult to predict how a prostate cancer will progress. The individual patient and his physician must weigh the possibly deleterious effects of screening against the possible benefits.

For these two reasons, an accurate diagnosis is of utmost importance. The key to an accurate diagnosis with the highest chance of survival is early detection.

Symptoms

Early prostate cancer usually produces no symptoms and is discovered during a routine physical examination either by a positive digital rectum exam or an elevated PSA level which may lead to a biopsy. Once symptoms appear, they often resemble those of benign prostatic hyperplasia (BPH). This can be dangerous, because non-cancerous enlargement of the prostate is common in men over 40, and difficulty with urination may be attributed to aging rather than disease.

Men experiencing the symptoms of BPH should see their physician immediately for a thorough examination.

Signs and symptoms for prostate cancer include the following:

- Blood in the urine or semen

- Frequent urination, especially at night

- Inability to urinate

- Nagging pain or stiffness in the back, hips, upper thighs or pelvis

- Pain during ejaculation

- Pain or burning during urination

- Weak or interrupted urinary flow

Changing your diet
could lower your risk.

Studies show a strong connection between consumption of saturated fat and red meat and increased rates of prostate cancer diagnosis and mortality.

More recent studies have found a connection between obesity and incidence of prostate cancer. Doctors now know PSA levels are more difficult to detect in obese men due to a PSA that is diluted by increased blood volume from excess weight.

Researchers found that a diet low in fat, high in vegetables and fruit, and avoiding high energy intake, excessive meat, and excessive dairy products and calcium intake may be helpful in preventing prostate cancer, and for patients diagnosed with prostate cancer.

Specifically, consumption of tomatoes, cauliflower, broccoli, green tea, and vitamins including Vitamin E and selenium seemed to propose a decreased risk of prostate cancer.

Consumption of highly processed or charcoaled meats, dairy products, and fats seemed to be correlated with prostate cancer.

Coffee: Consumption of six or more cups of coffee a day lowered the risk of being diagnosed with prostate cancer by 19%. The risk of developing aggressive prostate cancer was reduced by 41%. The more coffee you drink, the better the results (This is not proven by the ACS - only by health studies).

"Although not conclusive, results suggest that general dietary modification has a beneficial effect on the prevention of prostate cancer," the authors conclude. "In patients with prostate cancer, dietary therapy allows patients to be an active participant in their treatment."

Turmeric (Curcuma longa) a spice, the active phytonutrient in turmeric, actually interferes with the growth of tumors. Other spices that can help are Cayenne pepper, Cinnamon, Ginger and Cumin.

I use all the spices listed. Turmeric in white meats, Cayenne in fish, stews, tomato-base dishes, Cinnamon roasted figs, Ginger in honey, lemon, line, scallions, soy sauce, carrots and fish. Cumin in meats, beans, lentils, rice, potatoes and Mexican foods.

I have lost over 80lbs, Yes it took me six months, but I feel great now. Have more energy, better sleep, no more big stomach, Good overall health and 6-inches off my waist.

Exercise

- ❖ Another reason to exercise? Men who exercise at even moderate levels may have a lower risk of prostate cancer than sedentary men, a new study suggests.
- ❖ Exercise has been shown to have numerous health benefits, but studies have come to conflicting conclusions as to whether a lower risk of prostate cancer is one of them.

- ❖ The latest study, researchers found that among 190 men who underwent biopsies to detect possible prostate cancer, those who regularly exercised were less likely to be diagnosed with the disease.
- ❖ Men who exercised moderately -- the equivalent of three or more hours of brisk walking per week -- were two-thirds less likely than their sedentary counterparts to have prostate cancer.
- ❖ What's more, among men who did have cancer, those who reported as little as one hour of walking per week were less likely to have aggressive, faster-growing cancer.

Have you been treated with radioactive seeds or another form of radiation therapy?

Did you have unexpected side effects, pain or other problems after treatment? I want to hear from you. Please join the discussion and tell me about your experiences with your treatment or radiation therapy for cancer.

Sometimes radioactive treatments for cancer damage healthy body parts. Involving radioactive seed implants used to treat men with prostate cancer.

Many people who undergo external radiation therapy develop skin problem during their treatment that may continue after treatment has ended.

What is a PSA Test?

The PSA test is a simple blood test that can detect prostate cancer five to ten years before it becomes clinically evident.

The Institute recommends for men to keep track of their PSA level, as any one reading is not as significant as the "trend over time." We believe there isn't a "normal" PSA level, as the number may change due to a number of factors. One of the biggest influencing factors is age because the prostate grows as men mature, which, in turn, creates a higher PSA level.

For an accurate PSA reading, men should avoid:

- Sexual activity 48 hours prior to taking a test

- Excessive bike riding or lengthy car rides.

- Finally, never take a PSA test for two weeks after a digital rectal exam, or six to eight weeks after a TRUS or a biopsy. Any procedures dealing with the prostate—whether non-invasive or minimally invasive—will increase PSA levels.

Patients should have a TRUS done if the PSA level is more than 2.5 ng/ml or the digital rectal examination is abnormal, regardless of the PSA level. For high risk men, a TRUS examination is recommended if their PSA level is over 2.0 ng/ml.

Dr. Duke Bahn, one of the world's leading practitioners in the study and treatment of prostate cancer, is the Medical Director of the Institute.

Dr. Bahn has personally established a referral network of medical professionals—both locally and nationwide—that includes urologists, radiation oncologists, medical oncologists and psychologists devoted to the overall care of patients suffering from this disease.

Although we recognize that the following is not a complete list of every available option, it does present the seven most common approaches to addressing prostate cancer.

Active Surveillance

Watching cancer without treatment has long been a standard approach in the very elderly. However, today there are logical reasons to consider that Active Surveillance in good risk patents might be a safe and acceptable approach.

Cryotherapy

The controlled freezing of the prostate gland in order to destroy both the cancerous and surrounding tissue. It is done under sophisticated intra-operative ultrasound guidance.

Focal Cryotherapy

This provides an alternative to Active Surveillance for those patients who do not want to just watch their cancer and yet are not comfortable with any of the more invasive treatment options.

Brachytherapy (Seed Implantation)

Brachytherapy is a form of radiation in which tiny pellets containing radioactive material are implanted directly into the tumor-containing prostate, usually under ultrasound guidance.

Radiation Therapy

Using a CT Scan that creates a three dimensional image of the prostate area, doctors can specifically focus the radiation beam to target the entire tumor while sparing the surrounding normal tissue.

Surgical Treatment

Surgical Treatment, also referred to as a radical prostatectomy, is the removal of the prostate and seminal vesicles with open surgery. Recent developments in the field of surgical robotics have ushered in a new era of minimally invasive surgery that now challenges conventional open surgery. (da Vinci Laproscopic Radical Prostatectomy).

Hormone (Androgen) Deprivation Therapy

This treatment uses medications to suppress male hormone production from the body, based on the fact that the male hormone androgen is responsible for tumor growth.

Common skin problems that occur as a result of radiation therapy include:

- itchiness

- redness or sunburn-like appearance

- dryness

- general irritation

- skin may appear tan

These side effects occur in the area being exposed to radiation. People may also lose hair in the area being treated.

Tips for Managing Skin Irritation

During Radiation Therapy

[2]Radiation therapy is the medical use of high-energy beams of radiation targeted to kill cancer cells. Through a series of successive treatments, focused radiation damages cells that are in the path of the beam. Cancer cells are actively growing and replicating leaving them more vulnerable to radiation damage.

And because cancer cells are not as well-organized as healthy cells they are less able to repair the damage and recover. Thus, cancer cells are more easily destroyed by radiation, while healthy, normal cells repair themselves and survive. This is why radiation is such an effective cancer treatment.

One of the most uncomfortable side effects of radiation therapy is the reaction of the skin in the area being treated.

Similar to a sunburn the skin may react with a mild to moderate pink color, or redness accompanied by itching , burning, soreness, and possible peeling. Miaderm Radiation Relief Lotion soothes injured skin as well as helps to enhance the natural healing process and restore smooth, healthy skin without interfering with cancer treatment. end of [2]

[3]Miaderm Radiation Relief Lotion was developed by Radiation Oncologists with patient safety and comfort in mind.

Where can you buy Miaderm?
You can call the toll free number 877-642-7727 end of [3]

You also may try:
Using warm water and a mild soap to cleanse area during bathing. Baby soap is gentle enough.
Do not use scented perfumes, lotions, or creams on the treated area unless directed by a doctor.
Do not apply any cream two hours before or immediately after therapy unless directed by a doctor.
Do not wear tight fitting clothing around the treatment area. It may rub against the area causing irritation.
Avoid exposing the treated area to the sun or use tanning salons.
Avoid scratching the skin even if itchy.

Report any skin problems to your doctor. He or she may be able to prescribe an ointment or cream to reduce discomfort.

The chances of getting Prostate Cancer

The chances of getting prostate cancer are one in three if you have just one close relative (father or brother) with the disease.

There are no noticeable symptoms of prostate cancer while it is still in the early stages. This is why screening is so critical.

Every man age 45 or over should resolve to be screened annually. African-American men or those with a family history of the disease should start annual screening at 40.

The prostate gland is part of the male reproductive system; it produces fluid for semen. The prostate is about the same size and shape as a walnut, and sits in front of the rectum and below the bladder, where it surrounds the urethra that carries urine out from the bladder.

There are three ways that cancer spreads in the body.

The three ways that cancer spreads in the body are:

1. Through tissue. Cancer invades the surrounding normal tissue.

2. Through the lymph system. Cancer invades the lymph system and travels through the lymph vessels to other places in the body.

3. Through the blood. Cancer invades the veins and capillaries and travels through the blood to other places in the body.

WHAT IS PROSTATE CANCER?

Normally, cells grow and divide in an orderly way. Sometimes this normal process can go wrong. If abnormal cells continue to divide, they can form cancer tumors. Prostate cancer tends to occur in the cells lining the prostate. Its growth is usually slow and supported by male hormones.

Prostate cancer cells can spread to other parts of the body. There are no noticeable symptoms of prostate cancer while it is still in the early stages, which is why screening is so critical.

In more advanced stages, symptoms may include difficult or frequent urination, blood in the urine or bone pain.

EARLY DETECTION

Before early detection through PSA screening, only 1 in 4 prostate cancer cases were found while still in the early stages. With the widespread use of screening, about 9 out of 10 cases are now found early – giving men a fighting chance.

Nearly 100% of men diagnosed with prostate cancer while it is still in the early stages are still alive 5 years from diagnosis*. Of men diagnosed in the late stages of the disease, 33.4% survive 5 years*.

Screening for prostate cancer involves a simple blood test and a physical exam. It takes about 10 minutes and is covered by health insurance and Medicare in many states.

Obesity is a significant predictor of prostate cancer severity. Men with a body mass index over 32.5 have about 1/3 greater risk of dying from prostate cancer. Research shows high cholesterol levels are strongly associated with advanced prostate cancer.

Vitamin E, selenium, soy, green tea, tofu, tomatoes, and pomegranate appear to reduce the likelihood of getting cancer.

Additional studies are underway to confirm these findings, along with ongoing studies to discover and study additional cancer-fighting nutrients.

Men over 50 should take: a Nature Made Calcium Magnesium Zinc supplement and Vitamin D3. This helps promotes Bone, Colon and Breast Cancer.

Yes men can have Breast Cancer

TOOLS FOR EARLY DETECTION

The goal of early detection is to find the disease in its early stages when treatment is most likely to be effective. There are two widely used tests to aid in the early detection of prostate cancer.

Blood Test – PSA

This simple blood test measures the level of protein called prostate-specific antigen (PSA). Normally, PSA is found in the blood at very low levels. Elevated PSA readings can be a sign of prostate cancer; however, PSA levels can be elevated for reasons other than cancer.

Physical Exam – DRE The digital rectal exam (DRE) is a simple, safe and only slightly uncomfortable physical exam performed by your physician.

These exams are usually done together to increase the accuracy of diagnosis.

Although PSA will detect most high-risk cancers, there can be cancers that will be missed by this test and can be detected by the physical exam.

"The bottom line is there are no rules set in stone -- every man needs to talk to his doctor about when to start screening and how often, and in the event a cancer is suspected or diagnosed, they need to openly discuss the options of biopsy and ultimately, treatment," On your biopsy ask your doctor how many samples will be taken, your doctor should take at least two samples from each section (see page 38). A biopsy of just six samples one from each section in my opinion is not enough.

After prostate cancer has been diagnosed, tests are done to find out if cancer cells have spread within the prostate or to other parts of the body.

The process used to find out if cancer has spread within the prostate or to other parts of the body is called staging. The information gathered from the staging process determines the stage of the disease. It is important to know the stage in order to plan treatment. The following tests and procedures may be used in the staging process:

Radionuclide bone scan: A procedure to check if there are rapidly dividing cells, such as cancer cells, in the bone. A very small amount of radioactive material is injected into a vein and travels through the bloodstream. The radioactive material collects in the bones and is detected by a scanner.

What is a Biopsy?

Considered a minimally invasive procedure, a biopsy is the removal of a sample of tissue for the purpose of diagnosis. A biopsy is necessary because areas of inflammation or infection will often appear very similar to areas of cancer, and it is essential to absolutely rule out any possibility of cancer.

If a biopsy is performed, it will be a directed biopsy with tissue samples taken specifically from the noted abnormal areas. There is no predetermined number of tissue samples taken as each biopsy is a result of the individual findings on the ultrasound examination.

However, Dr. Bahn's and Dr. Silverman's experience coupled with the state-of-the-art technology used by the Institute, ensures that the tissue samples taken will be extremely accurate and be as few as possible.

Diagnostic accuracy is highly dependent on the skill and experience of the physician as well as the quality of equipment. Underestimation of the disease is the single-most common cause of selecting the wrong treatment option and as a result, leads to treatment failures. In previous studies, we reviewed 140 men with a known cancer diagnosis based on biopsies performed at other institutions that stated the cancer was confined within the prostate. All of the subjects had staging biopsies repeated by our staff. The result showed close to 30 percent of these men had cancer that was already outside of the prostate. In these cases, it was necessary to reconsider the treatment options and overall cancer management. Because of this, our mission continues to be the most accurate diagnosis possible.

Results of the biopsy are normally obtained within five to seven days. Dr. Bahn will personally call his patients with results as soon as he receives them.

"The male ego doesn't usually ever want to admit to having a problem. Men want to be macho and if they have a problem they just don't want to talk about it,"

Where to Get Screened

The Prostate Institute of America is located at:

Prostate Institute of America

168 N. Brent Street, Ventura, CA. 93003

Phone: 888-234-0004

Fax: 805-641-3965

Dr. Bahn's website: www.pioa.org

The Project to End Prostate Cancer operates the *Drive Against Prostate Cancer*, the only free national mobile screening program for prostate cancer I know of today.
Toll free: (888) 245-9455

As far as I know the only nationwide, mobile, free prostate cancer testing program. Email: info@zerocancer.org
http://www.zerocancer.org/index.html

Your primary care physician can do both the PSA test and physical examination. If you cannot afford a doctor's visit, call your local hospital or clinic to see if they offer a free screening program (most hospitals and some doctors do).

How Do I Decide on a Treatment?

Working with your doctor and other specialists, you can learn about your unique case, and discuss which treatment option will work best for you. Minimizing side effects and maintaining a high quality of life are serious factors to consider in the decision-making process. Potential side effects from treatment can include: Incontinence:

Prostatectomy or radiation therapy can disrupt the way the bladder holds urine by damaging the muscles that form the valves; treatment depends on severity, type and cause, and may include exercise, medicine, and restorative surgery.

Impotence: Erectile dysfunction (ED) is a common side effect following radical prostatectomy or radiation therapy; studies show that as many as 60-70 percent of men who have their nerves spared on both sides of the prostate will regain erections; 50-60 percent of men regain erections after radiation with the aid of ED drugs.

Pain: Treatment ranges from over-the counter pain killers and prescription narcotics to radiation treatment and acupuncture; treatment is also available for the pain and nausea caused by chemotherapy.

Depression

Depression: Occasional feelings of sadness, anger and anxiety are normal for people going through a major challenge like cancer.

If you are having trouble coping, don't be afraid to talk to your doctor; treatment can include counseling, medication, or a combination of the two.

If you Feel: Sadness throughout the day, nearly every day

Loss of interest in or enjoyment of your favorite activities

- ✓ Feelings of worthlessness
- ✓ Excessive or inappropriate feelings of guilt
- ✓ Thoughts of death or suicide
- ✓ Trouble making decisions
- ✓ Fatigue or lack of energy
- ✓ Sleeping too much or too little
- ✓ Change in appetite or weight
- ✓ Trouble concentrating
- ✓ Feelings of restlessness or being slowed down
- ✓ Thoughts about death or suicide are common in depression, and it's important to take such thoughts seriously.
- ✓ If you feel like giving up or as if you might hurt yourself, get help immediately:
- ✓ Call your doctor ,Go to the emergency room
- ✓ Call 911
- ✓ Call the National Suicide Prevention Helpline:
- ✓ 1-800-SUICIDE (1-800-784-2433)

Prostate Cancer is a tough opponent, but you can WIN by taking charge NOW!

Feeling Like a Man

After Prostate Cancer Treatment

Prostate cancer treatments often cause men to feel less like men

Urine leaks and a penis that won't get hard can cause a crisis in how a man feels about himself.

And, these may occur with prostate cancer treatment. Some men say they feel less manly, less independent.

Some say they don't even want to talk with women because they don't feel like "whole" men. They feel different.

The silence.

You might not hear much about this because men also think they shouldn't complain, show weakness, or get upset.

Men don't realize that it's normal to feel sad, angry, anxious, hopeless, and even grief-stricken at times. Prostate cancer treatments can be hard on a man's body and his mind.

You don't have to suffer in silence.

It helps if you can share your feelings with others close to you. You could try this:

• Talking with your partner, a close friend, or someone who has had prostate cancer

• Writing in a journal every day

• Joining a support group either in person or online

• Finding a counselor you are comfortable with Over time, you will gain a better sense of control and peace of mind.

The results and challenges of prostate cancer treatment vary from man to man. Some men come to terms with changes fairly quickly.

Others take much longer. Try the following tips and find out ways to manage your changes and challenges.

What can I do to help myself feel better?

Don't hide your feelings from yourself.

Don't pretend.

• Strong feelings are easier to manage when you admit to them. Being human, even being a male human, means having feelings. Learn to accept them, even the ones you don't "like."

• Keep in mind that feelings come and go. Even very powerful feelings lessen over time. Be patient with yourself.

• Find a way to share your feelings. You can use one of the ways listed above or other ways you have found helpful in the past.

Sharing feelings of sadness, anger, and stress decreases their power and may give you a better sense of control.

Find other men who have been through prostate cancer treatment.

Online is a good choice, talk to your doctor and ask if he/she know anyone you can speak too.

Look for a support group or for men you know who have had prostate cancer. Ask them how they coped with strong feelings, especially of not feeling like a "whole" man.

• Find a chat room on the internet to talk with other men recovering from cancer treatment.

See: http://www.lifeofhope109.org/

Keep in mind the things that make you feel like a man and continue to do them.

Ask yourself, "In what ways am I the same man as before the cancer?"

• Think about what you can still do that makes you feel like a man. Help others? Stay active and fit? Care for your home?

Be involved in work or a community group? If you have a partner, put effort into staying close and sexually active.

✓ Imagine sex as a new adventure.

✓ Think of erection aids and try to be playful.

✓ Be creative and experiment with new approaches. A sense of humor helps!

✓ Remember that your partner is learning too. Sharing feelings will help you and your partner feel closer.

✓ When you talk about your feelings, you will be more likely to work together to make sex good again.

It will take time to find new ways to pleasure one another. You might try planning sexy dates.

✓ When should I call or ask my doctor or nurse for help? Ask your doctor or nurse for a referral to a counselor when you:

✓ Feel depressed or anxious for more than 2 weeks, ...

✓ Feel that you can't get back your self-confidence as a man. You want a referral to a counselor who specializes in sexual problems Remember, asking for help doesn't mean you're weak. It means you're strong enough to admit that you can't do everything alone.

Prostate Cancer Vaccine

Is There Hope for a Prostate Cancer Vaccine?

[3]Numerous prostate cancer vaccines are in development and in various stages of clinical trials. A clinical trial is a rigorous scientific study of a potential therapy using human subjects. Clinical trials begin after scientists have accumulated enough data in lab studies to believe the therapy will be effective and not cause undue harm.

The effectiveness of cancer vaccines under development have improved significantly. Scientists are developing effective ways to deliver vaccines and combing vaccines with other immune system therapies seems to enhance the overall immune response. They've also identified characteristics of tumor-associated antigens, or markers that allow antibodies to recognize foreign invaders, leading to further improvements in vaccine research.

Prostate cancer vaccines, in particular, are advancing rapidly. This cancer often grows slowly, allowing vaccines sufficient time to generate an immune response. Furthermore, prostate cancer antigens direct the immune system to respond specifically to prostate cancer cells, sparing healthy tissue.

Here are updates on current prostate cancer vaccine activity.

The Food and Drug Administration approved a prostate cancer vaccine called Provenge, after the results of clinical trials provided evidence it prolonged men's lives on average four months and increased the three-year survival rate by 38 percent.

The potential vaccine POSTVAC-VF is in clinical trials. POSTVAC-VF increased mean overall survival rates for men by eight months more than men who took a placebo.

Scientists developed this vaccine based on the theory that the immune system fights cancer by directing it to attack specific targets on cells called Tumor Associated Antigens.

Currently, scientists are studying the potential of engineered measles viruses as a prostate cancer vaccine. In preliminary lab studies, they've found engineered measles viruses can effectively infect, replicate in and kill prostate cancer cells.

When researchers inject the virus directly into tumors, it significantly delays tumor growth.

Researchers are studying whether vaccines combined with hormone (androgen) deprivation therapy helps preventing recurrence by strengthening the patient's own immune system against prostate cancer. The vaccine may work by priming the immune system so when physicians add the hormone treatment, the vaccine is more effective.

You can visit www.clinicaltrials.gov to see what prostate cancer clinical trials are currently recruiting participants.

Provenge, a cancer vaccine, has demonstrated its ability to improve the survival of men with castrate resistant prostate cancer (CRPC). The developer, Dendreon, has submitted it latest clinical trial data to the FDA for approval.

They hope to have an approval by mid-year 2010.

Growth factors were thought to be potential targets for treating prostate cancer. Unfortunately, tests have proven the agents targeting these factors have been ineffective. Monoclonal antibodies to block IL-6 have been developed but the trials have been stopped due to excessive toxicity.

Calcitriol, a form of vitamin D3, has been combined with docetaxel (chemotherapy) in a clinical trial. However, it showed more deaths in the combination arm and the trial was stopped.

Anti-clusterin agents (clusterin is a protein associated with the clearance of cellular debris and apoptosis) in combination with docetaxel have shown improved survival in a randomized phase II trial.

Atrasentan, and denosumab attack the bone environment, a primary target for prostate cancer.

A)- Atrasentan, an endothelin receptor antagonist improved bone pain but did not improve survival.

B) – Denosumab is designed to target Rankel Ligand, a protein that acts as the primary signal to promote bone removal (Proper bone health requires bone removal and bone replacemrnt to be in balance).

A phase III trial involved 1,468 prostate cancer patients receiving hormone deprivation therapy (ADT),

who were randomized to receive either denosumab or a placebo every 6 months over a 36 month period. All subjects also received supplemental calcium and vitamin D. Of those taking the placebo, 3.9% experienced bone fractures during the 36 months, compared with 1.5% of those who received denosumab.

 The FDA delayed approval of denosumab in October 2009 because it wanted additional information about the drug.

ZD 4054 is a specific endothelian A inhibitor which when combined with docetaxel showed improved survival in phase II trials, but no difference in PSA response. Currently it is in phase III trials.

Docetaxel + bevacizumab (trade name Avastin), an anti-angiogenic agent, is being studied in CRPC and the results from a recently completed phase III trial is expected spring of 2010. Avastin recognizes and blocks vascular endothelial growth factors which serves as a chemical signal that stimulates the growth of new blood vessels to support tumors (angiogenesis).

Abiraterone and MDV 3100 are described as super androgen inhibitors by stopping androgen production in the testis, adrenals, and prostate. These agents are effective in chemotherapy naïve and resistant patients. A recently completed phase III trial evaluating abiraterone in CRPC who have failed docetaxel should report results soon.

Also called a TURP, this is a cystoscope [A Resectoscope Rather, which has 30 degree of viewing angle, along with Resectoscopy Sheath & Working Element] is passed up the urethra to the prostate, where the surrounding prostate tissue is excised.

This is a common operation for benign prostatic hyperplasia (BPH) and outcomes are excellent for a high percentage of these patients (80-90%). A more refined and safer operation is by means of a holmium(Nd:YAG) high powered "red" laser.

A related laser procedure for relief of prostatic obstruction utilizes a potassium titanyl phosphate(KTP) laser to vaporize the adenoma.

More recently the KTP laser has been supplanted by a higher power laser source based on a lithium triborate crystal, though it is still commonly referred to as a "Greenlight" or KTP procedure. The specific advantages of utilizing laser energy rather than a traditional electrosurgical TURP is a decrease in the relative bloodloss, elimination of the risk of TUR-syndrome, the ability to treat larger glands, as well as treating patients who are actively being treated with anti-coagulation therapy for unrelated diagnoses.

Getting the word out

While many men have never heard of male menopause, often their physicians are hesitant to bring up the issue because there are still so many unanswered questions about who would benefit from replacement therapy.

"I know men are interested in it and I know more men are showing up for a diagnosis and treatment.

You can just see that more prescriptions for testosterone are being given out. There is steady growth.

For now, most medical experts agree that only men over the age of 40 with symptoms of low testosterone should have a blood test and be screened.

The NIH has asked the Institute of Medicine to determine whether a large study on testosterone replacement therapy, similar to the Women's Health Initiative, is justified. Committee members at the IOM have been interviewing experts on testosterone therapy, including Morley, and a recommendation is expected later.

With all the different concepts on PSA testing and grading the Gleason score, ask your doctor which pathologist lab he/she uses to obtain your biopsy report.

Pathologist have their on unique way in analyzing Prostate Cancer Cells. No two pathologist analyze the same way, but they do follow a standard protocol in analyzing.

Don't be scared to check out the lab, its your right.

Briefs

The Type of Underwear you will need after the catheter is out.

Boxer Briefs or Briefs

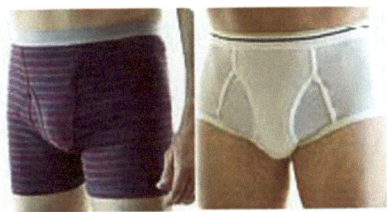

Be sure to bring these items with you when you go to have the catheter taken out. Don't forget to bring a few pads also.

You can purchase Underwear for Men at most Major Stores

Pads

You can purchase Pads for Men at most Major Stores

Pads for Men

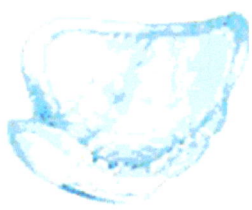

Pads for Men are a cup-shaped pad specifically designed to fit the aleanatomy. They are wider at the top and then taper down towards the bottom of the pad.

Ultra thin super absorbent design provides extra protection without extra bulk. Most are individually wrapped in a cloth-like pouch for discreet carrying.

1. Designed for Comfort: Soft outer cover with side barriers to prevent leaks.

2. Cup-Like Shape: Gives a close fit without extra bulk.

3. Adhesive strips ensure stay-put comfort when active.

How To Help Control your Urination After the Catheter is out.

1. Follow your doctors advice on Kegel Exercises for your system, do this regular during the day.

2. Go to the bathroom regular about every hour or so.

3. During Urination Try to stop your flow (5 sec).

4. Sit down on the toilet and work your stomach mussels like if you are having a bowl movement, this forces any urine out of your bladder.

5. After you feel you have a fairly good control over your bladder (this depends on the individual so be patent) try going without the pad during the day only, put your pad on at bedtime until your pad at night is Completely Dry.

6. Beware of things that make you dribble, like coughing, sneezing, passing gas and other things that puts pressure on you system. If you need to pass gas go to the bathroom and SIT!

7. The more you try to stimulate your penis the faster you will gain an ED. Foreplay with your partner, 5mg of Cialis, Pumps, Injections I suggest You Talk to your Urologist on this matter.

8. Even after you have control over your urination keep doing your exercises until you feel completely comfortable.. Note: you may have a stronger, heaver and faster flow during urination after you have your prostate removed. I know I do and many other men said the same.

9. Join a support group, at your local hospital or a online support group. You will get a lot of feed back on all the difference options.

10. On my studies I found Men over 45 should have a PSA test at least once a year. when a man turns 50, I suggest having a PAS test twice a year. It's a simple matter of just drawing a little blood for the PSA test. Early detection can improve your chances of successful treatment.

11. Note: After your biopsy you may have some blood in your semen, So wear protection the first few times when having sex. This is normal the first few times during ejaculation.

12. Keep doing you're your excises even after you have full control for at least 30 to 45 days. You need to know all your options…

When you have your Biopsy

The biopsy is basely pain free, the only thing you will feel is the injection to deaden the Prostate about 5 to 6 injections into the prostate, the injections may sting a little.

The biopsy itself is pain free, your Urologist takes 6 or 12 to 13 samples from the prostate. All you hear is a loud popping sound each time the doctor takes a sample.

Note: After your biopsy you may have some blood in your semen, So wear protection the first few times when having sex. This is normal the first few times during ejaculation.

This picture below shows the cancer area in the prostate

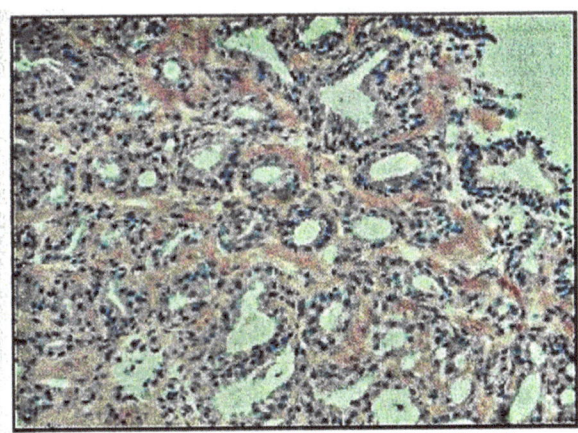

ADENOCARCINOMA RIGHT MID PROSTATE

This shows how the prostate biopsy is divided

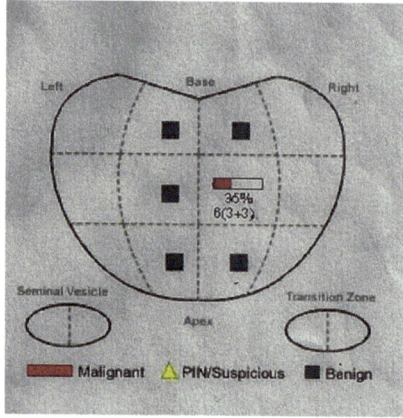

In some cases the biopsy will not show all the cancer in the prostate.

I also had cancer on the left side of 4 3+3. This is not uncommon!

If you have your prostate removed, the doctor will also send the Prostate to a lab to see if there were more cancer areas in your prostate.

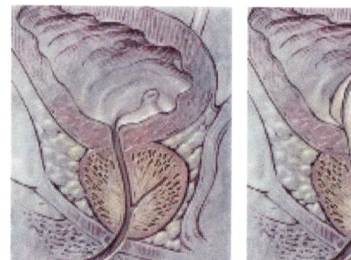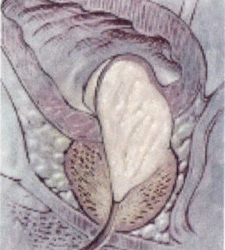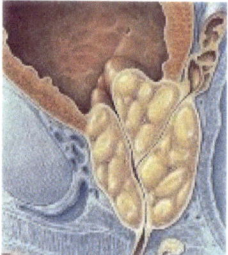

Normal Prostate-Inflamed Prostate-Enlarge Prostate

Know your prostate cancer

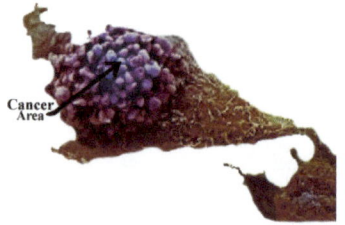

Cancer Area

Micrograph of prostate adenocarcinoma, acinar type, the most common type of prostate cancer.

Prostate Cancer Treatments: da Vinci Prostatectomy, which is a robotic-assisted laparoscopic surgery.

> Objectives:
> Surgeons remove the prostate and the cancer within it
> Time
> 1 to 2-day hospital stay, with a urinary catheter left in place for about 8 to 10 days

Know your prostate cancer treatment options

The prostate cancer treatment that is right for you will depend on many factors:

> Your age and expected life span
> Any other serious health conditions you may have
> How fast the cancer is growing
> How much the cancer has spread
> The likelihood that the treatment will cure your cancer
> Your feelings about the side effects or risks common with the treatment

Tumors that are still inside the prostate, radiation therapy, brachytherapy (seed implants), Precision Guidance for Radiation Therapy, cryotherapy and a surgery called radical prostatectomy are common treatment options.

Watchful waiting is also a treatment option. In this approach, no treatment is given until the tumor gets bigger. Watchful waiting may be the best choice for an older man with a slow growing tumor who has a higher risk of dying from something other than his prostate cancer.

Generally, cancer that has spread beyond the edge of the prostate and nearby tissue can't be cured with either radiation or surgery. It can be treated with hormone therapy or chemotherapy that slow the cancer's growth.

You may want to get a second opinion about the best treatment option for your situation, especially if there are several choices available to you. Prostate cancer is a complex disease, and doctors may differ in their opinions regarding the best treatment options. Speaking with doctors who specialize in different kinds of treatment, such as a urologist and a radiation oncologist, may be helpful for weighing your options.

Quick overview of prostate cancer treatment options

Surgery (Radical Prostatectomy)

Objectives:

Surgeons remove the prostate and the cancer within it

Time

2 to 3-day hospital stay, with a urinary catheter left in place for 2 to 3 weeks

External Beam Radiation Therapy

Objectives:

High-energy x-rays kill cancer cells

Time

15-minute treatments scheduled 5 days per week in an outpatient center over a period of 7 to 9 weeks

Precision Guidance for Radiation Therapy

Objectives:

Tumor tracking system guides the high-energy x-ray to precisely kill cancer cells without damaging healthy adjacent tissue.

Time

15-minute treatments scheduled 5 days per week in an outpatient center over a period of 7 to 9 weeks

(LDR) Brachytherapy - Low Dose Rate

Objectives:

Permanently implanted radioactive seeds deliver radiation to kill cancer cells

Time

After an outpatient procedure performed under anesthesia, radiation is delivered to the tumor over several weeks or months

(HDR) Brachytherapy - High Dose Rate

Objectives:

Radiation is delivered through temporary catheters in the prostate to kill cancer cells

Time

Radiation is delivered to the tumor in 1 or 2 sessions performed under anesthesia, typically requiring an overnight hospital stay

Watchful Waiting

Objectives:

Closely monitor the cancer without active treatment until the tumor grows or the cancer becomes aggressive.

Time

PSA blood test and digital rectal examination about every 3 to 6 months with repeat prostate biopsies, as needed

Hormone Therapy

Objectives:

Slow the growth of prostate cancer and shrink the size of the prostate

Time

Depends on the clinical situation and type of hormone therapy used

Chemotherapy

Objectives:

Slow the growth of prostate cancer and help reduce symptoms

Time

Depends on type and dose of drugs given by your doctor

High Intensive Focused Ultrasound for Prostate Cancer Therapy
HIFU

It's HIFU, High Intensity Focused Ultrasound, it cooks the cancer without any incisions or pain. The rate of incontinence is less than half of one percent, the ED rate is 20%-30%, but Cialis works for it.

The problem is it is not approved in the USA yet, it's been in use in Europe for 18 years with a 94% success rate. Japan posts a 97% success rate for low risk, and 67% for high risk. It is in clinical trials here, call 888-874-4384 for the Sonablate trial, or 866-650-4466 for Ablatherm trials. I understand that the trials are only concerned with curing the cancer, not saving quality of life....ask.

HIFU is a state-of-the-art technology utilizing the power of ultrasound to destroy deep seated prostate tissue without affecting the surrounding healthy tissue. The HIFU energy is focused sharply from the transducer surface to the targeted tissue in the prostate.

Temperature is elevated in the targeted tissue up to 90 degrees C within one second causing cell death.

The therapy consists of placing HIFU lesions (each requiring only a few seconds to create) side-by-side until the entire prostate gland has been "painted" with HIFU energy.

HIFU, readily available at affiliated International Treatment Centers in Mexico and in the Bahamas, is only approved by the FDA for investigational use within the United States.

Cryoablation of the prostate

By: Duke K. Bahn, M.D., Paul Silverman, M.D.1 & John C. Rewcastle, Ph.D.2

Dr. Bahn is certified by the American Board of Radiology and has served as the Clinical Associate Professor in radiation oncology at Wayne State University Medical College in Detroit , Michigan . He is a member of the American College of Radiology, the Radiology Society of North America, the Michigan Radiology Society, the California Radiological Society, the American College of Cryomedicine, the American Roentgen Ray Society, and the Society of Urologic Cryosurgeons.

Dr. Bahn is an active member of the Community Memorial Hospital Medical Staff and is currently the Director of the Prostate Institute of America.

1 Prostate Institute of America, Community Memorial Hospital, Ventura, California, USA

2 Department of Radiology, University of Calgary, Canada and Endocare, Inc., Irvine, California, USA. Duke K. Bahn, M.D.,

Paul Silverman, M.D.1 & John C. Rewcastle, Ph.D.2

1 Prostate Institute of America, Community Memorial Hospital, Ventura, California, USA

2 Department of Radiology, University of Calgary, Canada and Endocare, Inc., Irvine, California, USA
Carcinoma of the prostate is the most commonly diagnosed cancer in North America.

It accounts for one in three newly diagnosed cases and is the second most common cause of cancer death in males (1).

Widespread PSA screening has resulted in proportionally more men being diagnosed in the early stages of disease when a cure is possible.

However, the optimal management strategy for localized cancer remains unclear and is confounded by the myriad of available treatments and lack of objective comparisons between them. Radical prostatectomy and beam radiation therapy are historical standards of care and other treatments such as brachytherapy, conformal radiation therapy, intensity modulated radiation therapy and cryoablation have been added to the armamentarium used to battle prostate cancer

Technology: this is not your grandfather's cryo

Since the reintroduction of cryoablation in the early 1990s, several significant technical and procedural advances have occurred, including the development of vacuum insulated cryoprobes, the introduction of systematic temperature monitoring, the evolution of intraoperative treatment planning systems and, most recently, the development of a temperature feedback automated freezing system. Each of these innovations has been designed to assist the physician in learning and performing the three fundamental steps involved with prostate cryoablation:

1. planning the procedure based upon individual patient anatomy,

2. placing the cryoprobes and thermocouples within the prostate,

3. freezing the prostate such that the cancer is destroyed without compromising sensitive adjacent structures such as the external sphincter, urethra and rectum.

These technical advances can be used piecemeal, in concert, or not at all, depending on the experience and skill of the physician performing the procedure and individual patient anatomy.

Smaller Cryoprobes

Most published reports establishing prostate cryoablation as a therapy with durable safety and efficacy have been based on patients treated with blunt tipped 3.4 mm diameter cryoprobes. Insertion of cryoprobes of this size necessitates the use of a dilation system that results in the consumption of a significant amount of operating room time for the less experienced physician.

Cryoprobes 2.4 mm in diameter with vacuum insulated shafts are now available with thermal profiles nearly identical to those produced by 3.4 mm cryoprobes (< 1mm changes in isotherm locations).

Treatment planning

a. Placement logic

In-vivo human studies have shown that reaching a temperature of -40 °C on two successive freeze thaw cycles ensures ablation of prostate carcinoma tissue (2).

Therefore, prostate cryoablation is performed with the goal of exposing the entire gland to a temperature of -40 °C or lower while minimizing cold exposure of the rectum and external sphincter to avoid collateral damages. Determination of an optimal probe placement is a mathematical problem. The available planning algorithm utilizes the four accepted 'rules' of cryoprobe placement as reported by Ellis in 2002 (3):

1. Cryoprobes should not be placed more than 2.0 cm apart,

2. Cryoprobes should not be placed more than 1.0 cm from the margin of the prostate,

3. The distance between the urethra and any cryoprobe should not be less than 0.8 cm, and

4. The posterior cryoprobes should be placed such that their separation is less than twice the distance to the posterior capsule of the prostate.

b. Mapping patient anatomy and determining cryoprobe placement

An ultrasound transducer mounted to a stepper that is fixed in space relative to the patient is used to serially image the longitudinal plane of the prostate. Collected images are transferred to a treatment planning system. Image recognition software is used with the aid of anatomic reference points defined by the user to determine the geometric anatomy of the prostate, urethra and rectum.

Utilizing this information the system generates an optimization probe placement.

A brachytherapy like grid that allows for angled cryoprobe placement can be attached to the ultrasound stepper and used to assist with cryoprobe placement. Cryoprobes are inserted though the perineum and advanced to the base of the bladder in the sagittal plane.

The grid can be removed from the platform and the stepper and then the ultrasound probe can be used freehand, unobstructed by a stepper or grid.

Because the grid is lightweight plastic, it will not pull the probes out of the body when released from the platform. Experienced physicians may bypass this time consuming procedure and can place the cryoprobes by free hand, yet satisfying the basic "rules".

Systematic Temperature Monitoring

The fundamental advancement that sparked renewed interest in prostate cryoablation was the use of real time ultrasound to visualize cryoprobe placement and iceball growth.

Ultrasound, however, is not without limitation. Ice has an acoustic impedance much different that that of soft tissue. Consequently, nearly all the incident acoustic signal is reflected when the wave reaches the frozen/unfrozen interface. This allows for excellent visualization of the hyperechoic line representing the proximal iceball edge but the user is rendered blind to all distal anatomy as no signal is returned from structures within or beyond the iceball. Temperature monitoring is used to overcome this acoustic shadowing effect.

Prior to the commencement of the freezing process, thermocouples are placed at strategic locations within and around the prostate.

They are used to both ensure that adequately cold temperatures are reached within the prostate and that sensitive adjacent structures, namely the rectum and external sphincter are maintained at temperatures warm enough to ensure maintenance of their structural and functional integrity.

Automatic freezing

Keeping track of the power settings of six to eight cryoprobes, thermocouple temperature readings and progression of the iceball as visualized on ultrasound can be a daunting task for beginners.

As such, automatic freezing software allows targeted temperatures to be inputted by the user as been developed.

The physician selects the target temperature for each thermocouple.

Typically, this is –40 °C for the thermocouples placed in zones to ensure ablation and > 0 °C for those placed in sensitive structures to ensure their preservation.

All cryoprobes are controlled by a computer, which determines the optimal cryoprobe power settings based upon real time temperature feedback from the thermocouple tips. Freezing commences in an anterior to posterior manner to maximize transrectal ultrasound visualization.

If at any point during the procedure the temperature reading of any thermocouple placed in a sensitive structure drops below the safety margin set by the user, all probes stop freezing and begin to actively thaw to ensure no damage.

The freezing process must still be monitored carefully by the physician and can be overridden at any point allowing the physician to stop the freeze or continue to freeze manually controlling the cryoprobe power settings. Many experienced physicians do not utilize this automatic freezing technique. They can actually sculpture the ice to make an exact fit for the prostate, resulting in a complete ablation. It is indeed an art form.

Efficacy and Morbidity

In deciding what treatment is best for them, the individual patient in concert with his physician balances the perceived risks and benefits associated with each treatment option.

No therapy can guarantee a cure and unfortunately, no therapy can promise complete maintenance of quality of life. Many factors are taken into account when choosing a treatment including the stage and aggressiveness of the cancer, age, life expectancy, physical and sexual activity level and co-morbidities. The treatment decided upon is a balance of the patient's acceptance of cure probability, tolerance of potential morbidities and long-term quality of life impact.

Primary cryoablation

Randomized prospective clinical trials comparing the efficacies and morbidities of primary prostate cancer therapies are lacking.

As such, unflawed comparisons of different treatment modalities are complicated by comparisons of often retrospective, singleinstitution case studies with non-uniform patient selection. Further, definitions of biochemical failure (PSA based failure) vary from study to study.

That being said, comparisons looking at trends in efficacy and morbidity are certainly possible and are merited.

Fortunately, many institutions have reported outcomes following prostate cancer therapy with patients stratified according to risk group. This is done by reviewing three fundamental disease state measurements: stage, Gleason sum and PSA.

Each of these can be considered to be favorable or unfavorable. A favorable stage is T2a or less. Favorable Gleason sum and PSAs are < 7 and <10 ng/ml, respectively. Low risk disease has no unfavorable characteristics, moderate risk has one and high risk has two or three.

In 2003, Katz and Rewcastle presented an analysis of the literature based upon all studies published as full manuscripts in the peer reviewed literature over a 10 year period that reported five year Biochemical Disease Free Survival (BDFS) rates following definitive prostate cancer intervention (4). Although there wasn't consistency in the definition of BDFS, the analysis was intended to look for trends and was not designed to conclusively compare the different therapies.

Figures 1 through 3 show the published range of BDFS for each therapy observed five years following treatment for low, moderate and high risk prostate cancer, respectively.

Excellent local and systemic control is achieved with all therapies for low-risk disease.

Given the relative equivalence in efficacy, the treatment decision for this risk group should be based heavily on morbidity and quality of life factors.

Figures 2 and 3 compare the range of reported BDFS for patients with moderate and high-risk disease. Comparing with Figure 1, a drop in efficacy is observed for all therapies with increasing disease risk. However, the drop is not as substantial for cryoablation as it is for both surgical and radiation series.

Based on this comparison, the efficacy of cryosurgery appears to be at least equivalent to all forms of radiation therapy and surgery for moderate and high risk patients.

Another measure of efficacy is the positive biopsy rate which was also reviewed by Katz and Rewcastle(4).

The positive biopsy rates recently reported following cryoablation have been reported to be between 2 and 18%. The mean follow up of these studies was 5.1 and 2 years, respectively. The positive biopsy rates reported in the literature for brachytherapy, conformal beam radiation, and external beam radiation tend to be higher.

Studies of brachytherapy found positive biopsies to range from 5-26%, with mean follow-up periods of 18 months to 10 years. One study reporting positive biopsy rates following conformal beam radiation found it to be 48% at a mean follow-up of > 30 months. Following external beam radiation therapy the rates ranged from 20%-71%, with a mean follow-up of 2-6.8 years.

However, positive biopsy rates following radiation therapy can be misleading as radiation protocols are continuously changing and these rates may reflect outmoded dosing strategies.

It can be concluded that the efficacy of cryoablation is at least equivalent to radical prostatectomy and all forms of radiation therapy. It also appears to be superior in the treatment of higher risk disease.

Katz and Rewcastle provided a hypothesis as to why this may be so. There are two fundamental shortcomings to the standard therapies that can limit their ability to effectively treat locally extensive or biologically aggressive prostate cancer: positive margins observed after radical prostatectomy and the preferential killing of lower Gleason grade cancer by radiation therapy. The ability of radical prostatectomy to cure prostate cancer is defined by its ability to remove all tumor cells. Following prostatectomy, positive surgical margin rates are observed in up to 40% of patients.

Lateral freeze beyond the capsule of the prostate is usually done during cryoablation in case there is microscopic capsular penetration by the tumor. Seminal vesicle freezing is also possible if tumor involvement is confirmed.

This decreases the probability of cancer remaining in the patient. The disease extent defines how aggressively the user freezes laterally.

Radiation therapy ablates tissue by damaging the nucleus of individual cells. The more aggressive the cancer is, the harder the cells are to kill.

Certainly any cell will be irreversibly damaged if exposed to enough radiation but the sensitivity of the anatomic neighborhood of the prostate limits the lifetime dose of radiation that can be delivered to the gland. Clinical results indicate that efficacy of radiation therapy declines significantly if a patient's Gleason score is greater than 7 or has an aneuploid tumor. In fact, if cancer recurs following a trial of radiation therapy it is often a more aggressive form, which indicates a preferential killing of less aggressive cells only to leave those that are more radioresistant.

Recently, Bahn and his colleague reported that the efficacy of cryoablation is independent to the ploidy. Cryoablation offers mechanical destruction of tissue by forming a lethal iceball and ischemic necrosis by interrupting the blood flow during the procedure.

Procedural and technical advances, along with increasing experience of individual physicians have resulted in a steady decline of cryoablation morbidity.

Urethrorectal fistula was a great concern during cryoablation. Of the three latest cryoablation studies (5-7), only one found rectal complications (Bahn et al with fistula < 0.1%). This is directly related to an increased use of temperature monitoring of the Denonvillier's fascia and improved ultrasound technology. Incontinence in the three studies ranged from 1.3% to 5.4% and rates of post operative impotence ranged from 82.4% to 100%.

Table 1 compares the different forms of rectal injury and their rates for the different therapies (4). Urinary morbidity among radical surgery patients included permanent incontinence in 7-52%, while urinary morbidity among brachytherapy and beam radiation patients included incontinence ranging from 0-19% and 0-15%, respectively.

Impotence occurred at a rate of 51-96% in radical surgery studies, and at a range of 50-61% and 14-66% in beam radiation and brachytherapy studies, respectively.

A three year prospective quality of life impact analysis is available following cryoablation (8). The authors administered two scales, the FACT-P, and the SNQ.

A return to pre-surgical functioning in all areas, with the exception of sexual functioning was observed one year post cryoablation. At three years, 47% of impotent men who were previously potent prior to the procedure returned to having intercourse with or without assistance. All other areas of functioning remained high. There was no delayed-onset morbidity associated with cryoablation. These results imply that post cryoablation quality of life is comparable, if not superior, to that of other treatments.

Salvage cryoablation

Radiation therapy is widely used to treat localized prostate cancer.

However, recurrence and residual disease have been recorded in 25% to 93% of radiation cases and the procedure may not be repeated (9). The unique characteristics of radioresistant prostate cancer leave patients with limited options if the disease does recur. Primary radiation therapy results in micro and macroscopic tissues changes that often result in the unfortunate situation of aggressive disease located in a challenging surgical environment.

Radial prostatectomy following failed radiation therapy can be performed with curative intent but is associated with significant morbidity. Hormonal therapy (androgen deprivation) may reduce tumor size and slow the growth but is ultimately not curative and is too associated with significant quality of life impact. Considering the limitations of these treatments, an alternative approach to cure recurrent prostate cancer with minimal morbidity is desired. Significant interest in the potential ability of cryoablation to fill this therapeutic void has resulted in much work in the past decade that has established cryoablation as the preferred therapy for localized radiorecurrent prostate cancer.

Comparing the outcomes of salvage cryoablation and salvage radical prostatectomy is limited to comparing similar reports. Again, no comparative trials exist. Table 2 lists the ranges of BDFS, rectal injury and incontinence as published in the literature. For both therapies, the efficacy is lower and morbidity higher than that when prostates that have not been irradiated are treated. Efficacies appear to be similar and a conclusion other than equivalence would be inappropriate.

The difference arises when one looks at the morbidity. Although statistical comparison would be ineffectual the differences are compelling: essentially five and ten fold reductions in rectal injury and incontinence rates, respectively.

Although patients are carefully assessed prior to salvage therapy, be it cryoablation or radical prostatectomy, occult metastatic disease remains a concern. Treatment failure is often thought to be due to micrometastatic disease overlooked in salvage therapy workup.

These micrometastatic cells, found most often in bone marrow or lymph nodes, spread concurrently with radiation treatment and being outside of the prostatic capsule, remain beyond the realm of any salvage prostate cancer treatment. Several studies have correlated an elevated Gleason score in the primary tumor with an increased prevalence of micrometastatic cells and reverse-transcription polymerase chain reaction amplification of PSA mRNA has been proven to characterize metastatic cell proliferation.

Cher et al. have found an association between androgen ablation and a reduced prevalence of metastatic cells that could be useful in adjuvant primary therapies (10).

A phenotypic characterization assay performed in addition to standard bone scans would detect distant metastases earlier and improve treatment plans in patients likely to have micrometastatic bone marrow or lymphatic cancers. It is plausible that patients who fail definitive salvage therapy may have an etiology based on preexisting extracapsular or systemic cancers. With more careful screening and patient work-up, the success of cryosurgery to fully ablate localized radioresistant cancer may be greater than reported.

Personal Experience

Dr. Bahn have published 7-year outcomes of 590 patients who underwent cryoablation as a primary prostate cancer therapy (5) and 59 patients who had the procedure following biopsy proven post radiation therapy recurrence (9). A summary of these results are contained in table 3. As a primary therapy the results are comparable or superior to the rates of efficacy of all conventional radiation therapy modalities for prostate cancer.

There are also other advantages to cryoablation in comparison to conventional prostate cancer therapies. The procedure is extremely well tolerated. Only a short hospital stay is required with most patients being discharged within 24 hours. Cryoablation provides hope for those patients with locally advanced prostate cancer due to its ability to ablate laterally outside the glandular margin. It is also possible to ablate the seminal vesicles allowing the treatment of stage T3 disease.

An interesting psychology is at play after the procedure. In terms of quality of life and continence specifically, patients tend to improve over time. This yields a patient who tends to be happier than one whose morbidity increases or quality of life decreases following the procedure as can occur after radiation therapy (regardless of delivery modality). Impotence post procedure was high in our series. This was not surprising as the average age was 71 years and many patients had aggressive and/or bulky disease.

Recent reports indicate that impotence post procedure may not be as high as once though when baseline and post procedure sexual function is objectively quantified. There are no known latent complications following cryoablation.

Dr. Bahn and Dr. Silverman believe that the results they and others have published will lead to a greater acceptance and utilization of cryoablation as a primary treatment option for localized prostate cancer.

Recurrent prostate cancer following definitive radiation therapy tends to be extremely aggressive and dangerous. They have found that salvage cryosurgery is a promising form of treatment and we routinely offer it to patients who have failed radiation therapy. Their 7-year data shows biochemical control rates comparable with salvage radical prostatectomy series.

The compelling case for salvage cryoablation is when one considers the morbidity associated with both procedures. Incontinence and rectal injury rates following salvage radical prostatectomy are significantly higher. Indeed some cryoablation series have been published with high incontinence and fistula rates but these should be considered historic and are not reflective of outcomes achieved with the modern procedure performed with advanced technology. Cryoablation is a curative therapy with acceptable morbidity for a very hard to manage patient population.

Dr. Bahn and Dr. Silverman, encourage physicians to follow patients treated with radiation therapy closely as there is a window of opportunity in which the disease is still localized and a cure is possible.

Conclusion:

Technical and procedural modifications of cryoablation have led to a procedure today that is very different than what is was ten years ago.

It is a minimally invasive procedure, requiring a short hospital stay, with most patients discharged within 24 hours. Modern cryoablation, as a definitive therapy for both primary and radiorecurrent prostate cancer, is associated with minimal morbidity and no known latent complications. In fact, quality of life seems to continually improve following the procedure.

Cryoablation should be considered as a viable option for any patient who has been diagnosed with localized prostate cancer. Like all other options, it is not best for everyone but certainly there is sufficient evidence that it should be considered by everyone.

Dr. Bahn and Dr. Silverman are World Renown Urologist - Surgeons, Men from all over the World come to them for treatment, they have treated 100's of men from all over the world and too many to count from North America.

Acknowledgement: Thanks to Current Oncology Reports for granting permission to reproduce figures 1-3 of this article.

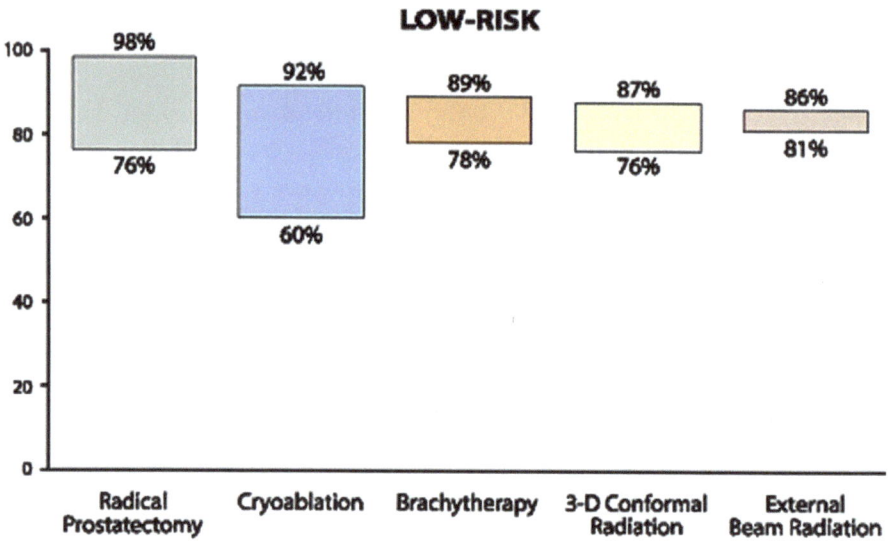

Figure 1: Comparison of Biochemical Disease Free rates for low-risk disease

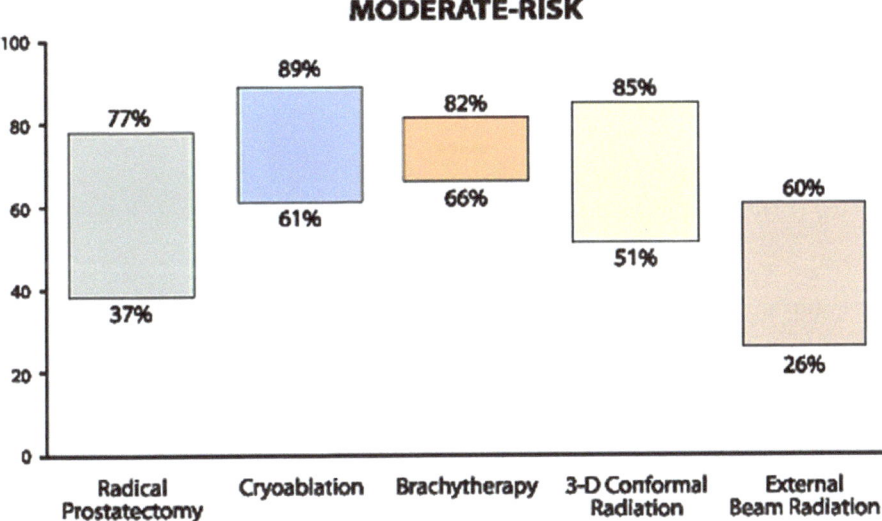

Figure 2: Comparison of Biochemical Disease Free rates for moderate-risk disease

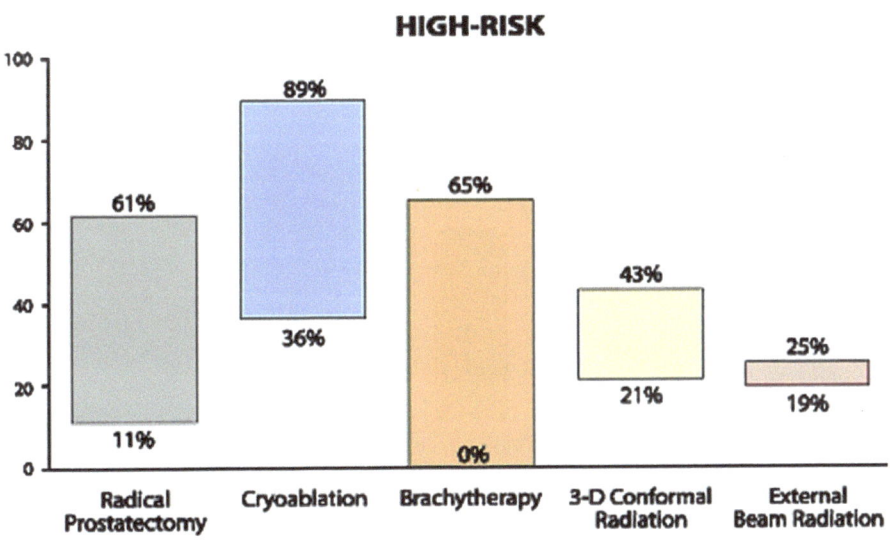

Figure 3: Comparison of Biochemical Disease Free rates for high-risk disease

Table 1: Comparison of the range of published rectal injury rates following definitive prostate cancer therapy

	Fistula	Urgency	Bleeding	Diarrhea
Radical Prostatectomy	1-3 %	6-16 %	1-3 %	6-19 %
Beam Radiation	19-43 %	13-17 %		12-42 %
Brachytherapy	0-3 %	4 –11 %		
Cryoablation	0-0.5 %			

Table 2: comparison of published ranges of BDFS, rectal injury and incontinence rates following salvage cryoablation and salvage radical prostatectomy

BDFS	59 – 69 %	30 – 82 %
Rectal injury	0 – 2 %	1 – 10 %
Incontinence	4.3 – 7.9 %	0 – 64 %

Table 3: Summary of our personal cryoablation experience

	Primary	Salvage
n	590	59
median PSA	6.8 ng/ml	5.6 ng/ml
median Gleason	7	7
median stage	T2b	T2c
ASTRO	89%	N/R
7-year PSA < 1.0	76%	69%
BDFS PSA < 0.5	62%	59%
Negative biopsy rate	87%	100%
Incontinence	4.3%	8%
[1]Fistula	<0.1%	3.4% (early in experience)
Impotence	95%	N/R

Reference List

(1) Jemal A, Tiwari RC, Murray T, Ghafoor A, Samuels A, Ward E, Feuer EJ, Thun MJ. Cancer statistics, 2004. CA Cancer J Clin 2004 January;54(1):8-29.

(2) Larson TR, Rrobertson DW, Corica A, Bostwick DG. In vivo interstitial temperature mapping of the human prostate during cryosurgery with correlation to histopathologic outcomes. Urology 2000 April;55(4):547-52.

(3) Ellis DS. Cryosurgery as primary treatment for localized prostate cancer: a community hospital experience. Urology 2002 August;60(2 Suppl 1):34-9.

(4) Katz AE, Rewcastle JC. The current and potential role of cryoablation as a primary therapy for localized prostate cancer. Curr Oncol Rep 2003 May;5(3):231-8.

(5) Bahn DK, Lee F, Badalament R, Kumar A, Greski J, Chernick M. Targeted cryoablation of the prostate: 7-year outcomes in the primary treatment of prostate cancer. Urology 2002 August;60(2 Suppl 1):3-11.

(6) Long JP, Bahn D, Lee F, Shinohara K, Chinn DO, Macaluso JN, Jr. Five-year retrospective, multi-institutional pooled analysis of cancer-related outcomes after cryosurgical ablation of the prostate. Urology 2001 March;57(3):518-23.

(7) Donnelly BJ, Saliken JC, Ernst DS, li-Ridha N, Brasher PM, Robinson JW, Rewcastle JC. Prospective trial of cryosurgical ablation of the prostate: five-year results. Urology 2002 October;60(4):645-9.

(8) Robinson JW, Donnelly BJ, Saliken JC, Weber BA, Ernst S, Rewcastle JC. Quality of life and sexuality of men with prostate cancer 3 years after cryosurgery. Urology 2002 August;60(2 Suppl 1):12-8.

(9) [1]Bahn DK, Lee F, Silverman P, Bahn E, Badalament R, Kumar A, Greski J, Rewcastle JC. Salvage cryosurgery for recurrent prostate cancer after radiation therapy: a seven-year follow-up.
Clin Prostate Cancer 2003 September;2(2):111-4.

(10) Cher ML, de Oliveira JG, Beaman AA, Nemeth JA, Hussain M, Wood DP, Jr. Cellular proliferation and prevalence of micrometastatic cells in the bone marrow of patients with clinically localized prostate cancer. Clin Cancer Res 1999 Septembe;5(9):2421-5.

Lifetime Risk

Based on rates from 2009, 17% of men born today will be diagnosed with cancer of the prostate at some time during their lifetime. This number can also be expressed as 1 in 6 men will be diagnosed with cancer of the prostate during their lifetime. These statistics are called the lifetime risk of developing cancer. Sometimes it is more useful to look at the probability of developing X cancer of the prostate between two age groups.

For example, 8.08% of men will develop cancer of the prostate between their 50th and 70th birthdays.

Removing the Cancerous Prostate

Removal of the cancerous prostate gland and certain surrounding structures is known as a radical prostatectomy.

In the United States, 91% of prostate cancer diagnoses are estimated to be clinically localized (confined to the prostate with no regional lymph node or distant metastasis, also referred to as stages T1 or T2) when first detected.

1. Because the entire prostate gland is removed with radical prostatectomy, the major potential benefit of this procedure is a cancer cure in patients for whom the prostate cancer is truly localized.

Radical Prostatectomy

Patients should discuss radical prostatectomy with their doctor to determine if they are an appropriate candidate.

The two potential side effects that most concern patients considering a radical prostatectomy are incontinence and inability to achieve erections.

Today, most patients are candidates for nerve-sparing radical prostatectomies when the cancer is detected early, and preventing nerve damage may significantly minimize the potential side effects of incontinence and impotence.

The vast majority of patients that undergo a radical prostatectomy see a return of urinary continence and sexual function after a recovery period post-surgery, though there is no guarantee that these benefits will apply for every patient.

The length of this recovery period depends on a variety of factors and patients should openly discuss what recovery they should individually expect with their doctor.

Types of Prostatectomy

Approaches to this procedure include traditional open surgery, conventional laparoscopic surgery or *da Vinci* Prostatectomy, which is a robotic-assisted laparoscopic surgery.

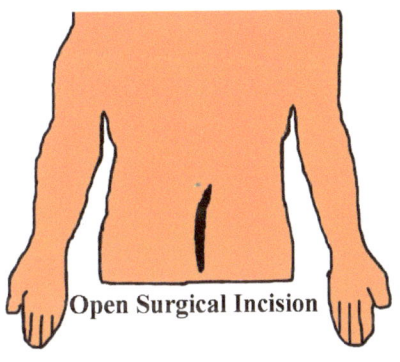
Open Surgical Incision

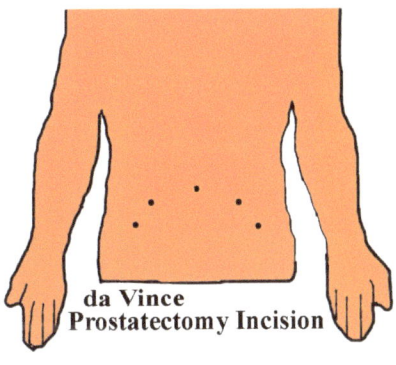
da Vince
Prostatectomy Incision

This picture is on my surgery

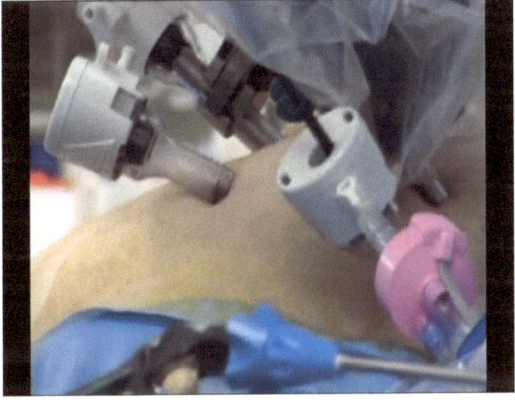

The da Vince Robotic at work

Dr. Paul D. Silverman at the Controls

Jerry's Recovery

1. Oct 28, 2009 Had the da Vinci Robotic Surgery at 1:10 P.M.

2. In recovery for one hour and 15 minutes.

3. Went to my room at 7:30 P.M.

4. I was Alert and Enjoyed my visitors of Family and Friends.

5. Went home on Friday morning about 10:00 A.M.

6. I had to wear the catheter for 8 1/2 days, but it was not bad at all, A little different when going to the bathroom but no big deal.

7. My Dr. removed the catheter at 9:30 A.M on Friday Nov 6, 2009 and the staples from my incisions.

8. I wore a pad day and night till Nov 19, 2009. Then I went all days wearing no Pad during the day, but did put a pad on at bedtime.

9. On Nov 23, No Pads Day or Night! I have full control over my urination.

10. I'm fully recovered and doing all my routines as before.

11. Don't rush your recovery, you may feel great but take your time and let your body heal.

12. Keep doing you're your excises even after you have full control for at least 30 - 45 days.

A Question a friend ask me:

Does the da Vince robotic surgery you had remove the prostrate ? I don't remember being offered that option but then again my Dr. thought I shouldn't even consider removing my prostate at 56. I had 5 weeks of external radiation followed by radiation pellets in the prostrate.
This has caused untold amounts of lost sleep due to pain/incontinence and very frequent urination 30 to 40 times a day/night. I can't leave the house without "traveling pants". I've even been surprised by uncontrollable bowel movements at times. You're so right about research. You really can't do too much. So many people I talked to before my treatment decision made radiation implants sound like a walk in the park.

My Dr's also seem surprised by my ongoing symptoms. I would also recommend avoiding here say. Talk to the guy that had the treatment.

Another problem came up with the external beam radiation I did in the first quarter of this year.....my legs and knees are very weak and sore, cannot do any real exercise.

My regular Doctor thinks it may be as a result of the radiation I took affecting the nerves in my lower back!

My Opinion and my answer back

Yes I had the Prostate removed, and my Dr, saved my nerves (ED=erection) Even at 56 your doctor should have told you all the treatments available plus give you some literature.

The seed implants can cause the prostate to turn to muss, and the 5 weeks of external radiation didn't help none.

Two Functions of the Bladder

The bladder is made of two types of muscles: the detrusor, a muscular sac that stores urine and squeezes to empty, and the sphincter, a circular group of muscles at the bottom or neck of the bladder that automatically stay contracted to hold the urine in and automatically relax when the detrusor contracts to let the urine into the urethra. A third group of muscles below the bladder (pelvic floor muscles) can contract to keep urine back.

Bladder training and related strategies

Bladder training consists of exercises for strengthening and coordinating muscles of the bladder and urethra, and may help the control of urination. These techniques teach us to anticipate the need to urinate and prevent urination when away from a toilet. Techniques that may help nighttime incontinence include:

- ✓ Determining bladder capacity

- ✓ Stretching the bladder (delaying urinating)

- ✓ Drinking less fluid before sleeping

- ✓ Developing routines for waking up

Unfortunately, none of the above has demonstrated proven success, but I know they do help!

Techniques that may help daytime and night time incontinence include:

- ✓ Urinating on a schedule, such as every 2 hours (this is called timed voiding) during daytime hours.
- ✓ Avoiding caffeine or other foods or drinks at night, that may contribute to a man's urinary function.
- ✓ Following suggestions for healthy urination, such as relaxing muscles and taking your time
- ✓ Do your Kegel Exercises as directed by your doctor.

I think that many men (including some I have known very well) might indeed prefer to die than to live with the permanent loss of sexual function. Sexuality isn't a trivial or an unimportant thing for some people.

Their wives or partners very likely wouldn't agree with those men that their lives would not be worth living without sex–I completely understand why the wife or partner would say "I want you alive, no matter what." But many men DO feel that their sexuality is so crucial a part of who they are that they'd rather die several years sooner than live an extended life without sexual function.

We can tell them they're "wrong" to feel that way, but that's not helpful; the point is that, given how many men in fact do feel that way, they need to be informed fully and carefully about exactly what they're risking before they choose to have the surgery.

✓ Men need to set their pride aside and look at the whole picture.

✓ Men need to look for the future of their family (not sex) and be around for the long run.

✓ Men need to speak out about their personal feeling!

A prostate removal, or radical prostatectomy, is usually done only to stop prostate cancer from spreading.

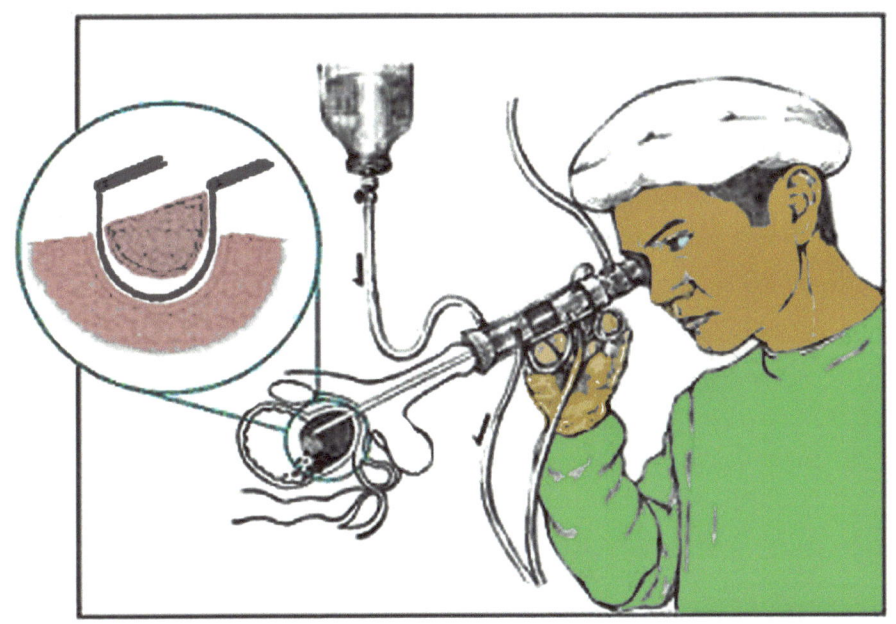

In TURP, a wire loop is used to cut away pieces of the prostate.

The Role of TRUS-Guided (Not Random) Biopsies in Determining the Internal and External Spread of PC

Dr. Fred Lee and Dr. Duke K. Bahn, M.D., published their data comparing sextant (random) biopsy proven PC data with our staging biopsy data on 110 men. All men came to us for a second opinion with known cancer. We performed TRUS with repeat staging biopsies on all of those men. (Seminars in Urologic Oncology, Vol 16, 1998, p 129-136.) The results were as follows:

➤ 26% of the Stage T1-T2 (tumor confined within the prostate) cancers defined by sextant biopsy were upstaged to T3-T4 (non-confined) by our staging biopsy technique.

➤ The Gleason sum was also higher in our staging biopsies.

➤ Perineural invasion was demonstrated in 52% of staging biopsies compared to 21% in sextant biopsies.

➤ Diagnosing unsuspected extracapsular extension and perineural invasion objectifies the choice of definitive treatment.

Information (Risk Factors) Needed from TRUS and Staging Biopsy

- ➢ What is the exact location of the tumor?
- ➢ What is the tumor size in the core by millimeters and dimension of the lesion TRUS?
- ➢ What is the Gleason grade? (If it is 7, what percentage is 4?)
- ➢ Is there a presence of perineural invasion (PC invading the nerve sheath within the prostate)?
- ➢ Is the tumor contained in the prostate or not (T1-2 or T3-4)?
- ➢ What is the ploidy of the tumor?

This information will provide the exact local staging of the cancer and will thereby help the physician and patient choose appropriately, a further staging work-up and decide on eventual treatment options.

Gleason Score	Rate of Cancer Growth
6 or Less	Average
3 + 4 = 7	Moderately Faster
4 + 3 = 7	Very Fast
8 - 10	Extremely Fast

State-of-the-Art Ultrasound Equipment

It is important to use a high-end, up-to-date ultrasound unit for an early detection and accurate staging biopsy.

Power Color Doppler ultrasound demonstrates all the blood flow patterns inside the prostate.

Usually, cancer tissue shows a higher blood flow (tumor neo-vascularity) than that of normal tissue. This capability will improve detection and actual tumor size measurement.

The newly developed Tissue Harmonic technology improves spatial resolution to permit visualization of smaller objects and improves contrast resolution to discern very subtle differences in grayscale. This is different from conventional ultrasound imaging, which sends out a burst of sound and listens for that burst to echo off structures in the body, (an echo that is usually weak and distorted).

The time it takes for the echo to return is proportional to the distance the sound wave travelled. In Tissue Harmonic technology, instead of listening for the same sound burst to return in the echo, the ultrasound equipment listens only for a sound burst at twice the transmitted frequency.

Good ultrasound evaluation with staging (strategic) biopsy may eliminate an unnecessary endo-rectal MRI study (that is still an imaging study without tissue confirmation).

Moreover, it will eliminate the "guesstimation" from random biopsies. Currently, we use the Hitachi EUB-6500 Ultrasound model.

Soon, there will be further developments in TRUS that will include contrast (IV form of micro-bubbles), enhanced Color Doppler, and three-dimensional imaging capability.

The Role of TRUS-Guided (Not Random) Biopsies in Determining the Internal and External Spread of PC

Dr. Fred Lee and Dr. Duke K. Bahn, M.D., published their data comparing sextant (random) biopsy proven PC data with our staging biopsy data on 110 men. All men came to us for a second opinion with known cancer. They performed TRUS with repeat staging biopsies on all of those men. (Seminars in Urologic Oncology, Vol 16, 1998, p 129-136.) The results were as follows:

> 26% of the Stage T1-T2 (tumor confined within the prostate) cancers defined by sextant biopsy were upstaged to T3-T4 (non-confined) by our staging biopsy technique.

> The Gleason sum was also higher in our staging biopsies.

> Perineural invasion was demonstrated in 52% of staging biopsies compared to 21% in sextant biopsies.

> Diagnosing unsuspected extracapsular extension and perineural invasion objectifies the choice of definitive treatment.

Current methods for determining confined PC for the individual patient are only guesstimations. The pathological outcomes for clinically confined PC have only a 50% probability of being correct. Today's patients seek answers through patient advocacy groups, Internet surfing, and scientific literature.

When one of our patients consults with the "specialists", he quickly surmises their uncertainty.

In our hands, the use of state-of-the-art TRUS with Color Doppler and Tissue Harmonic has helped us, and others, to resolve the uncertainty of whether a cancer is or is not confined, and what other risk factors they may have.

Then, and only then, do we more reliably predict a prognosis and guide our patients to those treatments that are most appropriate for them.

References

Lee F. Bahn D. The role of TRUS-guided biopsies for determination of internal and external spread of prostate cancer. Seminars in Uro Oncology 16: 129-136, 1998

Making the Decision to Biopsy

- Determine the gland volume with TRUS measurements: Gland Volume = [width (w) x height (h) x length (l) x 0.5]

- Predicted PSA = gland volume x 0.12

- Excess PSA = serum PSA – predicted PSA

- Expected tumor volume = excess PSA/2 (1 cm^3 of cancer produces near 2 ng/ml of PSA)

- To determine average tumor dimension (w + h + l)/3, use the $\sqrt[3]{}$ of expected tumor volume.

- Then search for a hypoechoic lesion of this size

Sonographic Evaluation

Because clinically relevant (>0.5 cm) PC is nearly always hypoechoic (black on ultrasound) compared with normal prostate tissue, we only biopsy lesions that are visible by ultrasound.

Depending on tumor architecture, the degree of hypoechogenicity (darkness on ultrasound) ranges from obvious (nodular) to subtle (infiltrative) changes. Thus, it is incumbent on the physician performing the examination to be familiar with the zonal anatomy and morphologic presentation of prostate cancer.

Cancers in the outer gland (peripheral zone and central zone) and inner gland (transition zone) have different sonographic appearances and biologic behavior, and our threshold that defines whether to biopsy varies depending on lesion size, location, and amount of excess PSA.

Outer Gland Cancers

Outer gland cancers have a greater propensity than inner gland cancers for extracapsular spread because they can escape easily through the area of anatomic weakness (entry of neurovascular bundle branches, seminal vesicles, and apex).

Fortunately, these tumors are easy to visualize because the background tissue is more homogeneous than that of the inner gland.

Most outer gland cancers originate laterally at the entrance of the neurovascular bundles. To visualize and sample this area, we have found it best to perform the scanning and biopsy in the transverse plane.

When targeting outer gland lesions, we first biopsy the lesion and than sample the accompanying neurovascular branches tangentially along a plane just external to the prostatic capsule. A finding of a tumor intermixed with fat definitively diagnoses histologic stage T3 cancer. When outer gland tumors extend to the midline, They perform a biopsy of the confluence of the seminal vesicle and trapezoid space of the apex. The base and apex of the gland in this area are always biopsied to aid in the evaluations of the internal spread of cancer.

Hypoechoic lesions of the outer gland should be pursued vigorously because they can escape when they are relatively small. For this reason, Dr. Bahn and Dr. Silverman generally perform a biopsy of the lesions we see on the ultrasound when excess PSA suggests that a 1cm lesion may be present (excess PSA greater 2ng/ml).

If we do not find lesions in the outer gland by ultrasound, we generally do not perform random biopsies. At this point, we shift our attention to the inner gland (transition zone).

Inner Gland Cancers

TRUS can detect cancers in the inner gland, though its sensitivity is less than that for the outer gland. If the excess PSA is 4 to 6 ng/ml and no lesion is found in the outer gland, on must carefully scan the inner gland for a homogeneous, poorly defined hypoechoic lesion. We focus on the sites of anatomic weakness of the inner gland, the anterior apex and the bladder neck. Color-flow Doppler and (lately)

Tissue Harmonic aid in the diagnosis of these more difficult-to-see inner gland cancers because most tumors larger than 1 cm have neovascularity (abundant vessel inside of tumor) that is easily identifiable with these new technologies.

Given the confusing heterogeneous nature of the transition zone, color-flow may be the only clue for the presence of cancer in a subtle hypoechoic lesion.

For the inner gland, we take a watchful waiting approach when: (1) gland volume is greater than 50 cm; (2) no suspicious lesion of the anterior apex or apex or bladder neck area is seen; (3) excess PSA is less than 4 to 6 ng/ml; and (4) there is no outer gland lesion. In general, inner gland cancers have less aggressive prognostic factors (Gleason score and DNA ploidy) than outer gland cancers and tend to be confined until they attain very large volumes.

Therefore, we feel that these cancers do not need to be pursued as aggressively as outer gland cancers. To ensure that we have not overlooked a significant tumor, we repeat serum PSA testing at 4- to 6-month intervals. Should an upward trend continue, we re-ultrasound.

Staging Biopsy Technique

The biopsy samples should include one sample from the middle of the lesion, and all routes of possible tumor escape, based on known sites of anatomic weakness. The positive neurovascular bundle biopsy has to include fat cells in contact with tumor cells or the invaded nerve sheath; a seminal vesicle biopsy should include pigmented epithelium (specific cell layer of seminal vesicle). Because the prostate gland does not contain fat, the presence of this tissue in the specimen confirms an extra prostatic invasion. We stain the rectal end of the tissue core with blue ink before sending it to the laboratory.

This will allow us to determine the exact location of the tumor—an inked end signifies an outer gland (peripheral zone) tumor and a non-inked end indicates an inner gland tumor (transition zone).

Robotic Prostatectomy Benefits

Robotic Prostatectomy Benefits – Short-Term and Long-Term

The cutting edge da Vinci Surgical System has revolutionized prostate cancer treatment with the advent of robotic prostate surgery, also known as robotic prostatectomy.

Benefits of this minimally invasive procedure are realized by both the surgeon, through enhanced precision and visualization, and the patient, in short-term and long-term recovery.

Robotic prostatectomy benefits may include:

- Quicker return to normal activity

- Shorter hospitalization – most go home the next day

- Reduced risk of incontinence and impotence

- Less blood loss

- Reduced pain – most patients don't even need narcotics after surgery

- Fewer complications

- Less scarring than traditional open surgery

- Less risk of infection

Robotic Radical Prostatectomy – Revolutionary Technology

Screening for prostate cancer has led to increased public awareness and early detection, as well as a decline in mortality rates. Robotic radical prostatectomy (robotic-assisted laparoscopic removal of the prostate gland) is also a contributing factor to these encouraging trends.

In addition, this state-of-the-art surgical procedure can offer the best chance for complete recovery. Wristed instrumentation, tremor filtration and 3D magnification aid the surgeon in performing one of the most demanding aspects of the procedure – nerve-sparing for preservation of post-operative sexual function and continence. Along with cancer control, these are key elements in follow-up for patients undergoing treatment.

Robotic Prostate Surgery – Is it Right for You?

How Robotic Prostatectomy Works

The da Vinci surgical system combines the incredible dexterity of robotics and the three-dimensional depth perception of computer technology,

a characteristic missing from traditional open and traditional laparoscopic surgery. da Vinci robotic procedures rely on a robotic arm designed with seven degrees of motion to replicate the dexterity of a surgeon's wrist.

The da Vinci instruments offer a three-dimensional operative field, higher magnification and enhanced wrist-like dexterity, allowing the surgeon to make microsurgical movements as if he was using his own hand, a distinct improvement over the limits of standard laparoscopic instruments or open surgery. During surgery, a special, high resolution camera displays the operating site at 10-15 times better than a human eye.

The image processing is real time, clear, and bright. This 3-D Vision system uses filters to eliminate distortion and image fogging. Virtual 3-D images make it possible to perform minimally invasive surgery with precise surgical margins.

The da Vinci system allows the surgeon to operate while comfortably seated at an ergonomically designed console, and the instruments prevent the surgeon's hands from tiring.

Sex Guidelines After Prostate Removal:

Wait at least 4 weeks to engage in sex

The sensation of your climax is unaltered, but there will be no ejaculation

The return of erectile function varies from days, weeks and up to 12 months after surgery.

What Men Don't Want To Talk About

What is your Prostate

A donut-shaped gland the size and shape of a walnut that surrounds the upper portion of the male urethra. Its main function is to produce part of the fluid that makes up semen.

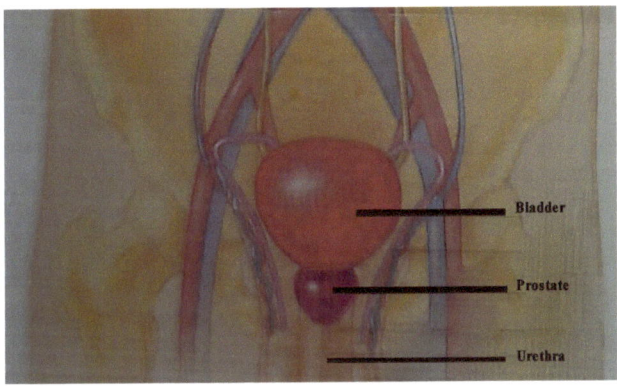

The American Cancer Society's most recent estimates for prostate cancer in the United States are for 2010:

192,280 new cases of prostate cancer

27,360 deaths from prostate cancer

Prostate cancer is the most common type of cancer found in American men, other than skin cancer. Prostate cancer is the second leading cause of cancer death in men. (Lung cancer is the first.) One man in 5 will get prostate cancer during his lifetime. And one man in 35 will die of this disease.

More than 2 million men in the United States who have had prostate cancer at some point are still alive today.

The death rate for prostate cancer is going down, and the disease is being found earlier, too.

The PSA test is a simple blood test to measure how much PSA (prostate specific antigen) a man has in his bloodstream at a given time.

The PSA test is the most effective test currently available for the early detection of prostate cancer.

My PSA was 6 (3+3) on the right side

6 (3+3) on the right, Gleason = 6 My PSA level now: 0.01

Prostate Cancer Symptoms

Early prostate cancer usually causes no symptoms. Often it is diagnosed during the workup for an elevated PSA noticed during a routine checkup.

It's highly advised to avoid sexual intercourse for 3 days prior to a PSA test because that affects the outcome of the test. Sometimes, however, prostate cancer does cause symptoms, often similar to those of diseases such as benign prostatic hypertrophy.

These include frequent urination, increased urination at night, difficulty starting and maintaining a steady stream of urine, blood in the urine, and painful urination. Prostate cancer is associated with urinary dysfunction as the prostate gland surrounds the prostatic urethra. Changes within the gland, therefore, directly affect urinary function.

Because the vas deferens deposits seminal fluid into the prostatic urethra,

and secretions from the prostate gland itself are included in semen content, prostate cancer may also cause problems with sexual function and performance, such as difficulty achieving erection or painful ejaculation.

Advanced prostate cancer can spread to other parts of the body, possibly causing additional symptoms. The most common symptom is bone pain, often in the vertebrae (bones of the spine), pelvis, or ribs. Spread of cancer into other bones such as the femur is usually to the proximal part of the bone.

Prostate cancer in the spine can also compress the spinal cord, causing leg weakness and urinary and fecal incontinence.

The cancer men don't talk about - prostate cancer

Senators Robert Dolc and Jesse Helms have it. So do Supreme Court Justices Harry A. Blackmun and John Paul Stevens. And 192,000 other American men get it each year.

They have the disease men don't talk about--cancer of the prostate. But men should be talking:

* Since 1985, rates have grown by six percent a year.

* It's the most common non-skin cancer among men, accounting for one out of every four men's cancers.

* It kills 100 American men each day. Only lung cancer is deadlier.

Sadly, many of those deaths can be chalked up to embarrassment.

If prostate cancer is detected early--using a simple test--the odds of surviving are more than 90 percent. Yet how many men do you know who have a yearly rectal exam?

So can we talk?

The prostate is a walnut-sized gland that straddles the urethra, the tube that drains urine from the bladder through the penis. It produces seminal fluid, which helps transport sperm.

"I was like most men, barely aware I even had one, much less aware it could develop into a life-threatening problem,"

THE FAT LINK

Eventually, one in 6 men will get prostate cancer. Those on the list:

* [4]Seniors. The older you are, the greater your chances . More than 80 percent of prostate tumors are diagnosed in men aged 65 or older.

Rates by Race Incidence

Race Ethnicity Male

All Races 159.3 per 100,000 men

White 153.0 per 100,000 men

Black 239.8 per 100,000 men

Hispanic 133.4 per 100,000 men

American Indian/Alaska Native 76.1 per 100,000 men

Asian/Pacific Islander 91.1 per 100,000 men

* African-Americans. American blacks have the highest rate of prostate cancer in the world. The culprit might be their slightly higher levels of testosterone, a harmone that stimulates the growth of prostate tumors.

Family history. Having a father or brother with prostate cancer more than doubles your risk.

* Race. African-American men are more likely to get prostate cancer than Caucasians, and the cancer is usually more advanced when discovered.

African-American men and men with a family history of prostate cancer usually begin prostate cancer screening at an earlier age than Caucasian men who do not have prostate cancer in their family history.

Prostatitis. Unlike most prostate problems, prostatitis — an infection of the prostate — occurs more often in young and middle-aged men. Only five percent to 10 percent of men develop prostatitis in their lifetime.

* If your family has a history of prostate cancer. A man has a much greater chance of developing prostate cancer if his father or a brother had it, particularly before age 65.

* People who eat diets high in fat (especially animal fat). "Populations that eat larger amounts of fat have strikingly higher rates of prostate cancer," says Curtis Mettlin, chief of epidemiology research at Roswell Park Memorial Institute in Buffalo, New York.

* Men in the United States, for example, eat large amounts of animal fat and have high death rates from prostate cancer. Greeks, on the other hand, eat about half as much animal fat as we do and are half as likely to die of prostate cancer.

[1] But it's not all nationality that makes the difference. It's also the environment.

Native-born Japanese who leave their country (where prostate cancer death rates are low) and move to Hawaii (where they're high) are three times more likely to die of prostate cancer than those who remain in Japan.

[2] "Differences in diet are the only way to explain why some countries have higher rates of prostate cancer than others," says Ernst Wynder, president of the American Health Foundation.

Studies that compare groups of people who live in the same country but who have different eating habits strengthen the link between fat and prostate cancer.

For example, Seventh-day Adventists who reported consuming the most meat, milk, cheese, and eggs were more than three times as likely to die of prostate cancer over the next 20 years than Seventh-day Adventists who said they ate the least amounts of those foods.

[3] And in Utah, men who recalled eating the most saturated fat were 80 percent more likely to have developed "aggressive" prostate cancer (the kind that spreads and is difficult to cure) than similar men who ate the least saturated fat.

[4] Most studies point to meats and dairy products, but it's impossible to completely exonerate vegetable fats until scientists come up with an animal that develops a similar tumor)

(a "model"), so that they can compare one fat's effects with another's.

How can fat affect the prostate? Some researchers believe that it raises the levels of testosterone and other hormones, which could stimulate the prostate to grow--along with any cancer cells it may harbor. end of [4]

"I still eat a little meat now and then, But I don't fry, Just a little olive oil then I cover the pan and add a little water and steam cook."

I also cut out soda, Candy, Sweets and Fast foods

Its okay to have a candy bar or sweets now and then, but try to limit your intake, once a month, We all want something sweet now and then.

So far, researchers haven't found that people who eat diets rich in fruits and vegetables have a lower risk of prostate cancer--a link that exists for lung and colon cancer.

And while scientists have suggested other risk factors (untreated venereal disease or the occupational exposure to cadmium, for example), none have been well-substantiated.

"NURSE, THE GLOVE, PLEASE"

"If prostate cancer is detected while it's confined to the prostate, the odds of surviving are very good--up to 90 percent,".

But if it has escaped the gland's outer jacket, the survival rate over the next five years falls to about 45 percent. And if it has spread to the lymph nodes, to the bone, or through the bloodstream to other organs, the odds of survival fall to 15 to 20 percent.

The two most common ways to detect a tumor are:

* Digital Rectal exam. Most prostate tumors can be felt by a finger inserted in the rectum. This is the easiest and least expensive way.

It's also the most embarrassing. Less than half of all American men who should be routinely getting a rectal exam do so.

"Men are just not taking care of themselves by getting their yearly checkups,".

* PSA test. An ailing prostate secretes a substance called prostate-specific antigen (PSA).

In some cases, a PSA test can reveal the presence of a cancer that the doctor can't feel through a rectal exam.

High blood levels of PSA are also found in men suffering from prostatitis (an inflammation of the gland) or from benign prostatic hyperplasia, an enlargement of the prostate that afflicts many middle-aged and older men.

(The jury is still out on whether an enlarged prostate increases the chances of developing cancer.)

And normal PSA readings could occur even if a cancer were present. That's why the test is most often used along with a rectal exam.

Using the rectal exam, doctors manage to catch about 60 percent of prostate cancers before they spread. Throw in a PSA test and the number jumps to nearly 70 percent.

HIDE OR SEEK?

If a cancer is caught early--when it's still confined to the prostate--the standard treatments are surgery (to remove the gland) or prostate cryoablation , radiation and many other choices.

If it has spread beyond the prostate, then it usually can't be cured.

Instead, its growth can be slowed--and some of the discomfort it causes relieved--by radiation or by cutting the body's production of testosterone, either through drugs or removing the testicles.

"These treatments have their pluses and their minuses,"

Radiation or surgery to remove the prostate causes temporary or permanent impotence or incontinence about half the time.

Some researcher's and others don't endorse the American Cancer Society's recommendation that all men over 50 get an annual PSA test along with their rectal exam.

"The PSA test may identify many men with small, slow-growing cancers who will then want to be cured with treatments that may be more destructive than the tumors themselves,".

Others see no reason to wait, when a man can easily find out if he has prostate cancer. Then he can evaluate his options.

"Better to over-diagnose than under-diagnose. "because by the time we find 40 percent of these cancers, it's too late to cure them."

"I'm one of the many men who consider themselves living proof that early detection can mean a healthy future. Please get routine checkups, and don't neglect to have your doctor check your PSA, blood pressure and your cholesterol for prostate disease. It could save your life." A bonus to having your cholesterol measured is that it is a good indicator of how your lifestyle changes are working.

The Four Stages for Prostate Cancer

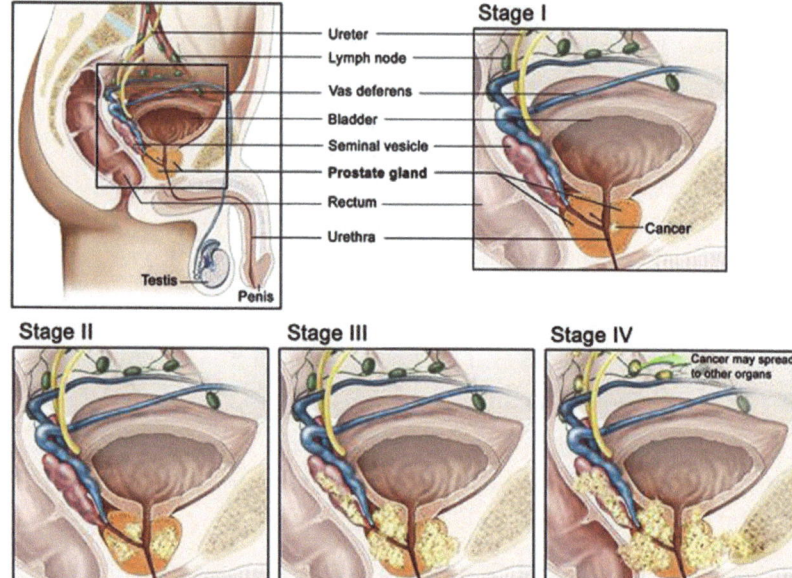

Know Your Stage! Ask your doctor What Stage you are in

Stage I

[4]Cancer that began in the prostate and is found in the prostate only. It cannot be felt during a digital rectal exam and is not visible by imaging. It is usually found during surgery for other reasons, such as benign prostatic hyperplasia (a condition in which an overgrowth of prostate tissue occurs). The Gleason score (a number that describes how abnormal the cells look under a microscope) is low.

The Gleason score is low. Stage I prostate cancer may also be called stage A1 prostate cancer.

Stage II

In stage II, cancer is more advanced than in stage I, but has not spread outside the prostate. The Gleason score can range from 2-10. Stage II prostate cancer may also be called stage A2, stage B1, or stage B2 prostate cancer.

Stage III

In stage III, cancer has spread beyond the outer layer of the prostate to nearby tissues. Cancer may be found in the seminal vesicles. The Gleason score can range from 2-10. Stage III prostate cancer may also be called stage C prostate cancer.

Stage IV

In stage IV, cancer has metastasized (spread) to lymph nodes near or far from the prostate or to other parts of the body, such as the bladder, rectum, bones, liver, or lungs. Metastatic prostate cancer often spreads to the bones. The Gleason score can range from 2-10.

Stage IV prostate cancer may also be called stage D1 or stage D2 prostate cancer.

Treatment Options by Stage

Current clinical trials for each treatment section. For some types or stages of cancer, there may not be any trials listed. Check with your doctor for clinical trials.

Stage I Prostate Cancer

Treatment of stage I prostate cancer may include the following:

Watchful waiting.

Radical prostatectomy, usually with pelvic lymphadenectomy, with or without radiation therapy after surgery. It may be possible to remove the prostate without damaging nerves that are necessary for an erection.

External-beam radiation therapy.

Implant radiation therapy.

A clinical trial of high-intensity focused ultrasound.

A clinical trial testing new types of treatment.

Check for U.S. clinical trials from NCI's PDQ Cancer Clinical Trials Registry that are now accepting patients with stage I prostate cancer. General information about clinical trials is available from the NCI Web site.

Stage II Prostate Cancer

Treatment of stage II prostate cancer may include the following:

Radical prostatectomy, with or without pelvic lymphadenectomy. Radiation therapy may be given after surgery. It may be possible to remove the prostate without damaging nerves that are necessary for an erection.

Watchful waiting.

External-beam radiation therapy with or without hormone therapy.

Implant radiation therapy.

A clinical trial of radiation therapy with or without hormone therapy.

A clinical trial of high-intensity focused ultrasound.

A clinical trial of ultrasound -guided cryosurgery.

A clinical trial of proton beam radiation therapy.

Clinical trials testing new types of treatment, such as hormone therapy followed by radical prostatectomy.

Check for U.S. clinical trials from NCI's PDQ Cancer Clinical Trials Registry that are now accepting patients with stage II prostate cancer.

For more specific results, refine the search by using other search features, such as the location of the trial, the type of treatment, or the name of the drug.

General information about clinical trials is available from the NCI

Stage III Prostate Cancer

Treatment of stage III prostate cancer may include the following:

External-beam radiation therapy with or without hormone therapy.

Hormone therapy.

Radical prostatectomy, with or without pelvic lymphadenectomy. Radiation therapy may be given after surgery.

Watchful waiting.

Radiation therapy, hormone therapy, or transurethral resection of the prostate as palliative therapy to relieve symptoms caused by the cancer.

A clinical trial of radiation therapy.

A clinical trial of ultrasound -guided cryosurgery.

A clinical trial testing new types of treatment.

Check for U.S. clinical trials from NCI's PDQ Cancer Clinical Trials Registry that are now accepting patients with stage III prostate cancer.

General information about clinical trials is available from the NCI Web site.

Stage IV Prostate Cancer

Treatment of stage IV prostate cancer may include the following:

Hormone therapy.

External-beam radiation therapy with or without hormone therapy.

Radiation therapy or transurethral resection of the prostate as palliative therapy to relieve symptoms caused by the cancer.

Watchful waiting.

A clinical trial of radical prostatectomy with orchiectomy.

Check for U.S. clinical trials from NCI's PDQ Cancer Clinical Trials Registry that are now accepting patients with stage IV prostate cancer.

For more specific results, refine the search by using other search features, such as the location of the trial, the type of treatment,

or the name of the drug. General information about clinical trials is available from the NIC website. end of 4

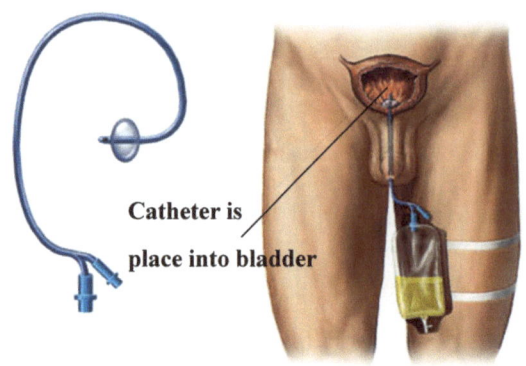

Catheter is

place into bladder

Web site: http://www.jmmotw.com/

Note: When you get home from the hospital, watch for excess blood lose and that your catheter does not leak.

Call you doctor ASAP if either appears to be excesses.

Not Getting A Good Night Sleep

Don't suffer another sleepless night. And try not to get discouraged if your current sleep aid is not working for you. Not all sleep aids are the same, so if one doesn't work for you, there are other options out there including over-the-counter (OTC) and prescription sleep aids. Of course, your healthcare professional is your best source for information; as he or she can take into account your unique medical history and lifestyle.

It's important to know that all medicines have side effects. If you experience any, or have any questions, you should speak to your healthcare professional.

A Quote from a friend

The seed implants may cause the prostate to turn mushy, and the five weeks of external radiation didn't help none.

This has caused untold amounts of lost sleep due to pain/incontinence and very frequent urination 30 to 40 times a day/night. I can't leave the house without "traveling pants". I've even been surprised by uncontrollable bowel movements at times.

Prescription sleep aids are approved by the Food & Drug Administration (FDA) to treat the symptoms of insomnia.

However, in some cases, people who have taken a prescription sleep aid have not found the good night's sleep they're looking for.

If this has happened to you, you should know that not all prescription sleep aids are the same. If one sleep aid is not working for you, another one may work better. Talk to your healthcare professional to find out what's right for you.

Some things to consider:

Try using a Condon Catheter "this could be your best way", Travel John's "men and women "and Pads for urination leaks after the catheter is out or other bladder control.

1. Know were the restrooms are located when traveling or commuting.

2. A Condon Catheter is very good when traveling or commuting.

3. Travel John's are also good "men and women".

4. Stress can be a trigger for overeating.

5. Anxiety, worry, depression about your condition can play a major role in your sleep habits.

6. Foods, When you are adventurous and experiment with new foods, you will eat more healthfully and most important, enjoy food more. Consuming lots of different flavors increases the number and type of nutrients you take in and boosts your feeling of satiety. You will feel full with less food in your stomach.

7. Clean Your Hands: Soap, wash your hands with warm-hot water and soap, "soap it off or eat it later.

8. Excise, Bicycling is a great way to excise at any age, the benefit of bicycling is low impact on the body.

9. Fat, to help trim belly fat, look at your diet. Avoiding refine carbohydrates (for example, sugar, white flour and products make with them; white potatoes; and pasta). Aim instead for the nutrient-and fiber-rich carbohydrates found in whole fruits and vegetables, whole grains and legumes.

10. Find a hobby you can do and enjoy.

11. Try a satisfying snack that fills you up with fewer calories.

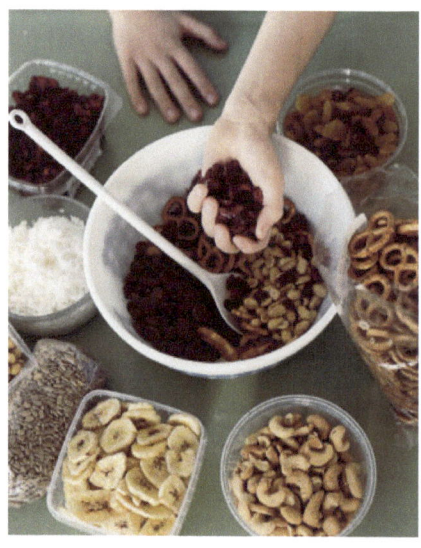

12. Take Care of yourself!

- ✓ **Eat a Healthy Breakfast**

- ✓ **Drink at Least 8 Glasses of Water**

- ✓ **Take a Good Quality Multiple Vitamin/Mineral**

- ✓ **Connect with Other People**

- ✓ **Express Your Emotions Appropriately**

- ✓ **Eat Fruits and Vegetables**

- ✓ **Spend at Least 30 Minutes Outdoors**

- ✓ **Do Something Physically Active**

- ✓ **Take Some Quiet Time for Yourself**

- ✓ **Keep Regular Sleep Hours**

- ✓ **Establish a Relationship with a Doctor You Can Trust**

✓ Have your thyroid glands check (this may cause you to be overweight and cause other problems)

Prescription sleep aids are approved to do different things. For example, some only help you fall asleep. Some prescription sleep aids are approved for short-term use only, so if you suffer from chronic insomnia, you may want to seek out a sleep aid that's not intended for short-term use only.

All prescription sleep aids contain risks of side effects.

I must say stress and worry can and will effect your sleep habits. (why I can't get a good night sleep after Prostate Surgery.)

I only had one night that I couldn't go to sleep and I was awake until 4:30 A.M. before I fell asleep for only 3 hours. Scene then I had no trouble. (I believe this was due to knowing I had Cancer)

I have always been a very positive person, I look at the glass and see it half full not half empty.

I feel this is a good way to look at our life in whole!

In general, I feel that surgery to completely remove the prostate is the best form of treatment and offers the best chance for cure. Now days, almost everyone prefers the da Vinci robotic surgery mainly because it is associated with less pain, shorter hospital stay, quicker time to recovery, less blood loss with less chance for needing a transfusion and get control over your body system a lot faster.
The incisions may be sore for a few days (the pain in your butt may last several weeks or more. (Not all men have this problem - butt.) I had no problem in this area.
I also believe Freezing (Cryotherapy)is another very good treatment.

Genetics

Genetic background may contribute to prostate cancer risk, as suggested by associations with race, family, and specific gene variants. In the United States, prostate cancer more commonly affects black men than white or Hispanic men, and is also more deadly in black men.

In contrast, the incidence and mortality rates for Hispanic men are one third lower than for non-Hispanic whites.

Men who have a brother or father with prostate cancer have twice the risk of developing prostate cancer. Studies of twins in Scandinavia suggest that forty percent of prostate cancer risk can be explained by inherited factors.

No single gene is responsible for prostate cancer; many different genes have been implicated. Mutations in *BRCA1* and *BRCA2*, important risk factors for ovarian cancer and breast cancer in women, have also been implicated in prostate cancer. Other linked genes include the "prostate cancer gene", HPC1, the androgen receptor, and the vitamin D receptor. The TEMPRSS2-ETS fusion gene exists in many prostate cancer cases and helps prostate cancer cells to survive and grow.

Determining the extent of prostate cancer is important for predicting the course of the disease and in choosing the best treatment. The TNM (tumor, nodes, metastasis) staging system is used to describe a cancer's clinical stage, or how far it has spread. This Health Alert provides an explanation of this important prostate cancer staging system.

The TNM system assigns a T number (T1 to T4) to describe the extent of the tumor as felt during a digital rectal exam (DRE). The N number (N0 to N1) indicates whether the cancer has spread to any lymph nodes, and the M number (M0 to M1) indicates the presence or absence of metastasis (spread to distant sites). The T and M designations are divided into subcategories (designated a, b, and c) that provide further detail on the extent of the cancer.

- T1a: Tumor found incidentally during surgery for benign prostatic hyperplasia (BPH) and is present in less than 5% of removed tissue

- T1b: Tumor found incidentally during BPH surgery but involves more than 5% of removed tissue

- T1c: Tumor found during needle biopsy for elevated PSA

T2: Tumor can be felt during DRE but is believed to be confined to the gland

- T2a: Tumor involves one half or less of one side of the prostate

- T2b: Tumor involves more than one half of one side but not both sides

- T2c: Tumor involves both sides of the prostate

T3: Tumor extends through the prostate capsule and may involve the seminal vesicles

- T3a: Tumor extends through the capsule but does not involve the seminal vesicles

- T3b: Tumor has spread to the seminal vesicles

T4: Tumor has invaded adjacent structures (other than the seminal vesicles), such as the bladder neck, rectum, or pelvic wall

NO: Cancer has not spread to any lymph nodes

N1: Cancer has spread to one or more regional lymph nodes (nodes in the pelvic region)

MO: No distant metastasis

M1: Distant metastasis

- M1a: Cancer has spread to distant lymph nodes

- M1b: Cancer has spread to the bones

- M1c: Cancer has spread to other organs, with or without bone involvement

Frequently Asked Questions

Q. [1]What is Minimally Invasive Surgery (MIS)?

A. MIS is surgery typically performed through small incisions, or operating ports, rather than large incisions, resulting in potentially shorter recovery times, fewer complications, reduced hospitalization costs and reduced trauma to the patient.

While MIS has become standard-of-care for particular surgical procedures, it has not been widely adopted for more complex or delicate procedures – for example,

prostatectomy and mitral valve repair. [1]Intuitive Surgical believes that surgeons have been slow to adopt MIS for complex procedures because they generally find that fine-tissue manipulation – such as dissecting and suturing – is more difficult than in open surgery. Intuitive Surgical's technology, however, enables the use of MIS techniques for complex procedures.

Q. [1]Why do we need a new way to do minimally invasive surgery?
A. Despite the widespread use of minimally invasive or laparoscopic surgery in today's hospitals, adoption of laparoscopic techniques, for the most part, has been limited to a few routine procedures.

This is due mostly to the limited capabilities of traditional laparoscopic technology, including standard video and rigid instruments, which surgeons must rely on to operate through small incisions.

In traditional open surgery, the physician makes a long incision and then widens it to access the anatomy.

In traditional minimally invasive surgery – which is widely used for routine procedures -- the surgeon operates using rigid, hand-operated instruments, which are passed through small incisions and views the anatomy on a standard video monitor.
 Neither this laparoscopic instrumentation nor the video monitor can provide the surgeon with the excellent visualization needed to perform complex surgery like valve repair or nerve-sparing prostatectomy.
Q. [1]What are the benefits of *da Vinci* Surgery compared with traditional methods of surgery?

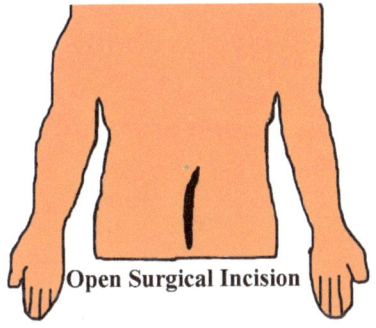

Open Surgical Incision

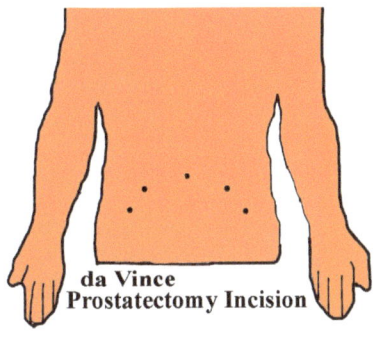

da Vince
Prostatectomy Incision

A. Some of the major benefits experienced by surgeons using the *da Vinci* Surgical System over traditional approaches have been greater surgical precision, increased range of motion, improved dexterity, enhanced visualization and improved access. Benefits experienced by patients may include a shorter hospital stay, less pain, less risk of infection, less blood loss, fewer transfusions, less scarring, faster recovery and a quicker return to normal daily activities.

None of these benefits can be guaranteed, as surgery is necessarily both patient- and procedure-specific.

Q. [1]Why can't surgeons perform complex procedures such as cardiac surgery through 1-2 cm ports today?

A. Complex procedures like cardiac surgery require an excellent view of the operative field and the ability to maneuver instruments within tight spaces with precision and control.

Surgeons historically have used invasive approaches like "open sternotomy" for heart surgery, which means splitting the breastbone and pulling back the ribs and typically results in a foot-long incision.

[1]This provides visibility and allows room for the surgeon to get his or her hands and instruments very close to the operative site, but results in significant pain, blood loss and a long recovery for patients. More recently, smaller incisions have been used to perform a variety of cardiac procedures. However, many cardiac surgeons feel the reduced access may limit visualization and may impede access to the operative field.

Q: [1]Where is the *da Vinci* Surgical System being used now?

A. Currently, The *da Vinci* Surgical System is being used in hundreds of locations worldwide, in major centers in the United States, Austria, Belgium, Canada, Denmark, France, Germany, Italy, India, Japan, the Netherlands, Romania, Saudi Arabia, Singapore, Sweden, Switzerland, United Kingdom, Australia and Turkey.

Q. [1] Has the *da Vinci* Surgical System been cleared by the FDA?

A. The U.S. Food and Drug Administration (FDA) has cleared the *da Vinci* Surgical System for a wide range of procedures.

Q: [1]Is *da Vinci* Surgery covered by insurance?

A. *da Vinci* Surgery is categorized as robot-assisted minimally invasive surgery, so any insurance that covers minimally invasive surgery generally covers *da Vinci* Surgery.

This is true for widely held insurance plans like Medicare. It is important to note that your coverage will depend on your plan and benefits package.

For specifics regarding reimbursement for *da Vinci* Surgery, or if you have been denied coverage, please call the Reimbursement Hotline at 1-888-868-4647 ext. 3128. From outside the United States, please call 33-1-39-04-26-90.

Q. [1]Will the *da Vinci* Surgical System make the surgeon unnecessary?

A. On the contrary, the *da Vinci* System enables surgeons to be more precise, advancing their technique and enhancing their capability in performing complex minimally invasive surgery.

The System replicates the surgeon's movements in real time. It cannot be programmed, nor can it make decisions on its own to move in any way or perform any type of surgical maneuver without the surgeon's input.

Q. [1]Is a surgeon using the *da Vinci* Surgical System operating in "virtual reality"?

A. Although seated at a console a few feet away from the patient, the surgeon views an actual image of the surgical field while operating in real-time, through tiny incisions, using miniaturized, wristed instruments.

At no time does the surgeon see a virtual image or program/command the system to perform any maneuver on its own/outside of the surgeon's direct, real-time control.

Q. [1]Is this telesurgery? Can you operate over long distances?

A. The *da Vinci* Surgical System can theoretically be used to operate over long distances.

This capability, however, is not the primary focus of the company and thus is not available with the current *da Vinci* Surgical System.

Q. [1]While using the *da Vinci* Surgical System, can the surgeon feel anything inside the patient's chest or abdomen?

A. The system relays some force feedback sensations from the operative field back to the surgeon throughout the procedure. This force feedback provides a substitute for tactile sensation and is augmented by the enhanced vision provided by the high-resolution 3D view.

Q: [1]What procedures have been performed using the *da Vinci* Surgical System? What additional procedures are possible?

A. The *da Vinci* System is a robotic surgical platform designed to enable complex procedures of all types to be performed

through 1-2 cm incisions or operating "ports."

To date, tens of thousands of procedures including general, urologic, gynecologic, thoracoscopic, and thoracoscopically-assisted cardiotomy procedures have been performed using the *da Vinci* Surgical System.

Q. [1]Why is it called the *da Vinci* Surgical System?

A. The product is called "*da Vinci*" in part because Leonardo *da Vinci* invented the first robot.

He also used unparalleled anatomical accuracy and three-dimensional details to bring his masterpieces to life. The *da Vinci* Surgical System similarly provides physicians with such enhanced detail and precision that the System can simulate an open surgical environment while allowing operation through tiny incisions.

[1]While clinical studies support the effectiveness of the *da Vinci* System when used in minimally invasive surgery, individual results may vary. end of [1]

Conclusion

Surgery with the *da Vinci* Surgical System may not be appropriate for every individual. Always ask your doctor about all treatment options, as well as their risks and benefits.

Today, there are a number of excellent treatment approaches that you 'may' or 'may not' be able to consider which may be dependent upon the type and stage of your cancer, meaning is it aggressive and or has it spread outside of the prostate gland, along with of course considering your age.

Most Doctors, Urologists and or Oncologists will recommend a couple to several options of which in 'their' professional opinion believe would best suite 'your case'.

Nonetheless, it is entirely up to 'you' to do some quick research on your own seeking out the 'advantages' and 'disadvantages' to the existing technologies in treatment for prostate cancer along with new technologies in treatment that may now be available.

But I would caution against dragging your research out too long in making a decision.
For 'your case', you will have to choose from the available choices, perhaps rather quickly and hopefully wisely. But more importantly with knowledge about the treatment; and of course based upon that knowledge you will have to choose the treatment that 'you' believe you will feel most comfortable with.

Remember when you provide another with comfort, when you lend a hand, or simply be there for someone who needs help, you transform the health of our country. Big change doesn't require a hero's effort.

Just one small act of kindness can make you a hero to someone else.
How will you Help?
Support Prostate Cancer

See: http://www.lifeofhope109.org/

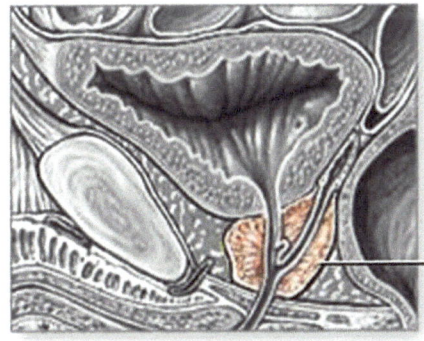
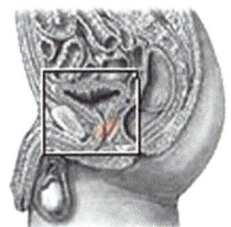

Normal prostate

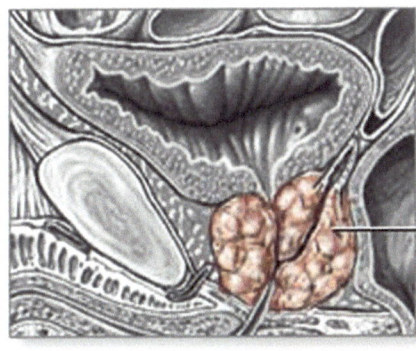

Prostate cancer

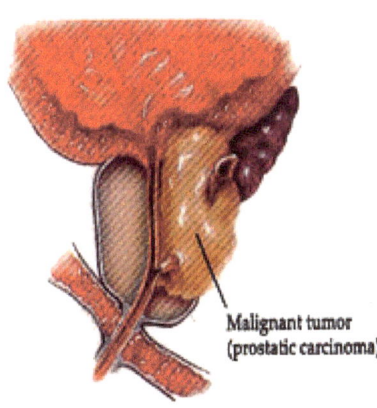

Malignant tumor
(prostatic carcinoma)

Treatment of prostate cancer varies depending on the stage of the cancer (i.e., spread) and may include surgical removal, radiation, chemotherapy, hormonal manipulation or a combination of these treatments.

You can ease the stress of illness by joining a support group whose members share common experiences and problems.
See: http://www.lifeofhope109.org/

One of the most effective ways of dealing with prostate cancer treatment is to remember:

- Be mentally prepared and healthy about your treatment. Determine what will help you accomplish this goal and do it! It may enhance your changes of a positive result.
- Remain Mentally Healthy
- I cannot stress this enough. Socialize, meditate, exercise, reduce stress, keep life in perspective, get a massage, go on a short trip, pursue your hobbies, laugh… do whatever you can to remain mentally healthy and happy. Its no secret that chronic mental depression may increase your risk of certain diseases. All avoid or treat depression!
- Be Realistic-Everything in Moderation. Be good to yourself. Do not become obsessive about anything you do.
- Alcohol in moderation
- Do not smoke
- When setting goals, ask yourself if you can implement the changes into your lifestyle on a permanent basis.
- Do you enjoy a thick, juicy steak once in a while? a hot dog or hamburger, etc. As mentioned previously, your mental attitude has a great deal to do with your overall health. If you are happy and content after eating your favorite food., then you should certainty partake once in a while!

In no way I'm suggesting any type of Treatment or Medications.
This is Your decision! Make it a wise one.

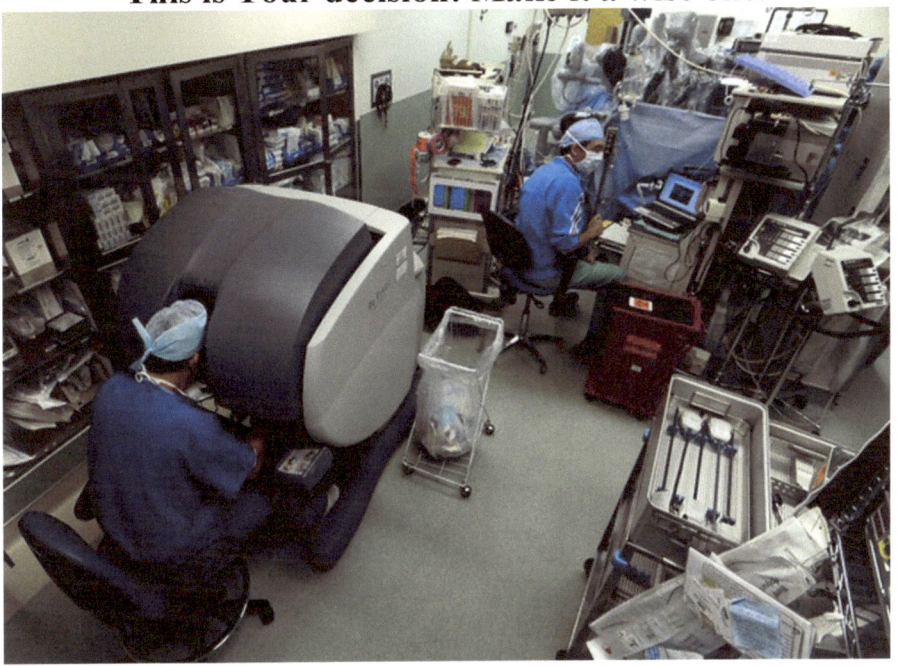

Dr Paul Silverman operating the da Vince Robotic

Keep the Life of Hope Alive!
Jerry L Mayers., CSAMS

Proceeds and Donations go to help men who can't
afford treatments or other help with Prostate Cancer.

Notes:

A Few Facts to Remember

Gleason: The lower the score, the better. A combined Gleason score of 10 is very bad (although there are still many treatments that doctors can offer men with high Gleason scores). Here's how the scores break down:

- Scores from 2 to 4 are very low on the cancer aggression scale.

- Scores from 5 to 6 are mildly aggressive.

- A score of 7 indicates that the cancer is moderately aggressive.

- Scores from 8 to 10 indicate that the cancer is highly aggressive.

Be honest (and unembarrassed) with your doctor.

Some symptoms are tough to talk about: sexual dysfunction, addictions, cancer, a rash "down there." Equally difficult to discuss are barriers, such as inability to read well or at all. Your honesty and directness can give your medical team the kind of information it needs to treat your needs.

For example, you may prefer watching a video, rather reading a pamphlet on a medical condition or prescription drug. Or, if you don't plan to fill a prescription because you can't afford it, your doctor needs to know.

Make sure you understand your doctor's orders.

Your physician may write out directions for you. You're likely to remember more if you jot down notes in your own handwriting. Consider writing a few words in response to each of these questions:

What is my main problem?

What do I need to do?

Why is it important for me to do this?

Make sure your doctor understands your thoughts and concerns

If possible bring someone with you to jot down notes

Sometimes we only hear what we want and don't get all the facts

Help Options : http://www.cancer.gov/help

http://www.lifeofhope109.org

References and Footnotes

[1]Footnotes: From http://www.prostatecancerdecision.org
[2]Footnotes: http://en.wikipedia.org/wiki/Prostate_cancer
[3]Footnotes: http://www.miaderm.com/
[4]Used by permission: Michigan Department of Community Health

All References and Footnotes use by Permission.

Author: Jerry L Mayers., CSAMS
Publish by: Life of Hope, http://www.lifeofhope109.org
Co Authors: Paul Silverman, M.D., Duke K. Bahn, M.D.

Dr. Bahn and Dr. Silverman are World Renown Urologist - Surgeons, Men from all over the World come to them for treatment and testing, they have treated 100's of men from all over the world and too many to count from North America.

The contents of the book, such as text, graphics, images, and other material contained in the book ("Content") are for informational purposes only. The Content is not intended to be a substitute for professional medical advice, diagnosis, or treatment. Always seek the advice of your physician or other qualified health provider with any questions you may have regarding a medical condition. Never disregard professional medical advice or delay in seeking it because of something you have read in the book!

If you think you may have a medical emergency, call your doctor or 911 immediately. Jerry Mayers does not recommend or endorse any specific tests, products, procedures, opinions, or other information that may be mentioned in the book. The book may contain health- or medical-related materials that are sexually explicit. If you find these materials offensive, you may not want to use this book.

The book and the Content are provided on an "as is" basis.

www.ingramcontent.com/pod-product-compliance
Lightning Source LLC
Chambersburg PA
CBHW040826180526
45159CB00001B/87